Health and Society in Early Modern Sweden

Health and Society in Early Modern Sweden

Edited by
Mari Eyice and
Charlotta Forss

Routledge
Taylor & Francis Group
LONDON AND NEW YORK

First published in 2024 by Amsterdam University Press Ltd.

Published 2025 by Routledge
4 Park Square, Milton Park, Abingdon, Oxon OX14 4RN
605 Third Avenue, New York, NY 10158

Routledge is an imprint of the Taylor & Francis Group, an informa business

ISBN: 9789463724296 (hbk)
ISBN: 9781041180784 (pbk)
ISBN: 9781003697220 (ebk)
NUR 680

Cover illustration: Jacob Elbfas, *Vädersolstavlan*, Storkyrkan, 1636. Oil on panel, 1630 × 1100 mm. Image: Göran Fredriksson, Stockholms Stadsmuseum. The painting portrays halos that were seen in Stockholm on April 20th 1535 and interpreted as portents. It is one of the earliest depictions of the city of Stockholm, seen from the South. This image is a copy made in 1636 by Jacob Elbfas, the original 16th century painting has been lost.

Cover design: Coördesign, Leiden

DOI: 10.5117/9789463724296

Table of Contents

List of Tables and Figures

Acknowledgements

The initial idea for this volume developed before health in society became everyone's top concern. Our project has since been formed by the Covid-19 pandemic and the reshaping of the academic and social interactions that followed from it. In January of 2020, we decided to collaborate on the topic of health and society in early modern Europe with scholars from around Europe. Once the pandemic had hit, our collaboration moved online and the extraordinary circumstances created an added sense of relevance and urgency to our enterprise. We would like to thank all of our colleagues for inspiring discussions during the initial phase of the project.

The chapters of this volume originate from a selection of the topics discussed in this initial phase. We developed our individual topic ideas collaboratively during online authors' sessions and presented the project at the Nordic Historians' meeting in Gothenburg in 2022, once the acute phase of the pandemic was over. We would like to thank everyone who participated in these events for their valuable comments and insights.

The book brings together ten authors who are affiliated with six different Swedish and Finnish universities and who work in the disciplines of history, history of science and ideas, and economic history. It has been a pleasure to work so closely with our colleagues throughout this project, and our work as editors has been made easy through your conscientious (and might we add, unusual and precious respect for deadlines. Your readings of each other's chapters at various stages of the work process have also been immensely valuable.

The whole project has been supported by the Department of History, Stockholm University, which we would like to thank for both practical support and for an inspiring research milieu. Karin Sennefelt suggested that we should publish an edited volume: thank you, Karin, for planting this seed. Alan Shima has done excellent work with language editing; all remaining errors are our own. Josef Eskhult has been extremely generous with his knowledge of the period and especially his insights on Georg Stiernhielm. Thank you, Josef, for your help and support!

We would like to thank our anonymous peer reviewer for valuable feedback. The editors at Amsterdam University Press have been enthusiastic and supportive throughout the whole work process: thank you, Wendy Turner and Shannon Cunningham. The editorial and research work for this volume have been carried out within the framework of our respective fellowships from the Swedish Research Council (2018-06765 and 2019-06278).

Finally, this volume is not only a product of academic labour but also a social endeavour. The editorial work has been carried out in between our respective parental leaves. We dedicate the book to Charlotta's son Axel and Mari's son Essa, who have been present at editorial meetings since their births, and for whom health in early modern society is mother's milk.

Mari Eyice and Charlotta Forss
Stockholm, July 2023

1. Meanings of Health in Early Modern Sweden

Charlotta Forss and Mari Eyice

Abstract

This introduction outlines a conceptual framework for analysing the historically situated nature of 'health.' While previous historical research has elucidated conceptions of illness as changeable over time, it is our contention that the meaning of health is often taken for granted. We examine the semantic field of 'health' (Swe. *hälsa*) and associated terms as they were used in early modern Sweden, showing health as a multifaceted concept with connotations to bodily and mental well-being, prosperity, politics, and religion alike. The individual chapters of the volume are situated in the broader account of early modern medicine, which highlights how a focus on a contextual understanding of health can inform the history of medicine and the broader account of early modern history.

Keywords: health, early modern history, social history of medicine, conceptual history

Introduction

In a poem entitled 'Hälse-Prijs' (Eng. 'In praise of health'), the Swedish seventeenth-century poet, scholar, and civil servant Georg Stiernhielm concluded that 'all is nothing, where health is not.'[1] To Stiernhielm, money, power, and worldly honours were all useless if he was not healthy. He explained that the person who is favoured with health 'lives happy in daily

1 Georg Stiernhielm, 'Hälse-Prijs.' On Stiernhielm, see Olsson, 'Georg Stiernhielm.' All translations into English in the introduction as well as in the chapters of the volume are the authors' own, unless otherwise stated.

Eyice, M. and C. Forss (eds.), *Health and Society in Early Modern Sweden*.
Taylor & Francis Group 2024
DOI 10.5117/9789463724296_CH01

joy, without sorrows,' until the day he falls ill, and then all good fortune is lost. To Stiernhielm's early modern reader, the poem 'Hälse-Prijs' would have been recognisable as a reference to the literary theme that fortune is fickle: it is well to remember that riches can vanish quickly.[2] To the modern reader, the poem appears to express familiar present-day sentiments regarding how highly we value good health. Yet this is also a poem that raises questions.

Stiernhielm was born in Dalecarlia in central Sweden in 1598, and he died in Stockholm in 1672. He lived in a time and a society without antiseptic surgery, extensive healthcare, welfare institutions, or modern notions of cleanliness, for that matter.[3] In light of this, we cannot assume that 'health' was understood the same way to Stiernhielm as it is conceptualised today.[4] What did Stiernhielm actually praise in his poem? When was a person considered healthy in early modern society, and when were they deemed ill? Furthermore, where did Stiernhielm understand good health to reside? In the poem, he speaks of bodily health and pain in one's foot or hand, but the poem also notes that an 'aching heart' and a miserable soul are the results of failed health. Clearly, health was not only a matter of bodily and mental well-being to Stiernhielm: instead, health affected, and was affected by, all facets of life.

The poem 'Hälse-Prijs' suggests that health was a complex matter in early modern society, yet it does not, despite its clever wordplay, elaborate on this complexity. However, where the poem leaves off, this volume continues the analysis. The chapters collected here take as their point of departure the conviction that the meaning and significance of health, as an idea and as a set of practices, has changed over time, and that it is an important task for historians to consider the historically specific notions and perceptions of health. More specifically, the volume consists of a set of case studies that explore health as a concept and a social practice in early modern Sweden.

2 This sentiment is also seen in Sparman, *Sundhetzens speghel*, 4. For an analysis of the fickle nature of fortune in learned discourse in early modern Sweden, see Savin, *Fortunas klädnader*; see also Nilsson, *Lyckans betydelse*, 218–219, for more popular views.

3 On early modern cleanliness, see North, *Sweet and Clean?*; Smith, *Clean*; Van Bavel, 'The Economic Origins of Cleanliness in the Dutch Golden Age.' On notions of health and cleanliness at the brink of modernity, see Annola, Drakman, and Ulväng eds., *Med tvål, vatten och flit*.

4 By posing open-ended questions concerning what 'good health' has meant historically, we do not negate the fact that there are very significant differences between and within societies with regards to access to healthcare today. On the contrary, it is our conviction that historical reflection can serve as a starting point for scrutiny of the conceptual categories we take for granted today. On conceptual history as a method to understand history, the present, and the ways in which historians approach both, see, e.g., Koselleck, *The Practice of Conceptual History*; Williams, *Keywords*.

These studies examine conceptions of healing in rural communities and matters of health in more densely populated areas. They explore topics such as how health was understood in Swedish society in relation to mental and physical disability, to food and leisure, and to the emergence of medical professions and changing notions of the body. Methodologically, they span between detailed biographical studies and analyses of long-term change.

Through this multilayered approach, the volume showcases how meanings of health were shaped by the specific cultural and social settings in which they were performed, and, conversely, how the meanings people attributed to health had a social significance beyond the realm of medicine. This approach addresses the social and cultural history of medicine, which, during recent decades, has brought attention to the importance of societal contexts for understanding past medical practice.[5]

However, the volume's contributors equally shed light on the opposite phenomenon, namely, how notions of health affected early modern society outside of the medical field, in the spheres of politics, consumer patterns, institutional developments, and social relations between people in their daily lives. While the history of medicine increasingly has taken societal developments into consideration when analysing medical history, there is still a tendency to think of the history of medicine as a separate field, and of understanding medical thought and practice as the end goal for historians of medicine. This is unfortunate. It is our starting point in this volume that the study of issues commonly understood as the traditional realm of the social history of medicine – including themes such as medical practitioners and their patients, the ailing and healing body, places of healing, and conceptions of health and illness – can lead to a better understanding of the broader narrative of early modern history.[6] Like the poet Stiernhielm, we approach health as an integral aspect of how people in early modern society lived their lives.

In this introduction, we present the two central themes of the volume – health and society – and discuss the respective chapters of the volume in relation to each of these themes. First, we consider how historians and

5 Swedish contributions include: Bergqvist, *Läkare och läkande*; Johannisson, *Medicinens öga*; Ling, *Kärringmedicin och vetenskap*. On broader European trends, see: Lindemann, *Medicine and Society in Early Modern Europe*; Gentilcore, *Food and Health in Early Modern Europe*, and the contributions in Kalof and Bynum, eds., *A Cultural History of the Human Body*; Carrera, ed., *Emotions and Health*; Ritchey and Strocchia, eds., *Gender, Health, and Healing*.

6 For an inspiring recontextualisation of health in early modern society, see, e.g., Van Bavel, 'The Economic Origins of Cleanliness.' For an early, formative approach to the social history of medicine, see Porter, 'The Patient's View.'

historians of medicine have previously understood 'health.' We emphasise the importance of contextualising health as a historical concept with changing meanings, and we point to areas where the individual chapters of this volume contribute to and enrich earlier research. Through this account, we begin to sketch how people in early modern Sweden understood health, a discussion that continues throughout the volume. Second, we survey the geographical area and the historical developments that constitute the framework of the volume, and place the contributions within this sociocultural context. While Sweden (including today's Finland) constitutes the main historical setting for the issues discussed here, this is a porous site in which people, ideas, and even institutions continually traverse and upend geographical as well as conceptual borders.

The early modern period, which constitutes the chronological framework for this volume, is likewise a porous construct.[7] The chapters stretch from the very beginning of the sixteenth century to the end of the nineteenth, tracing long-term development as well as highlighting moments of change. With this move, we have strived to go beyond modern periodisation to capture both continuities and breaks that otherwise tend to remain obscure. This is particularly relevant for the Swedish context where considerable scholarly attention in recent years has been devoted to – otherwise highly relevant – developments in the nineteenth and twentieth centuries.[8]

Highlighting the two central themes of the volume in relation to the individual chapters that make up the analysis, the introduction aims to provide a framework for considering historically situated meanings of health as a central aspect of early modern history, within and beyond the social history of medicine.

A conceptual history of 'health' in early modern Sweden

Health was a signifier of the good life in premodern societies. Within the concept of health resided ideas about 'tranquillity, happiness, and virtue,' according to Gideon Manning.[9] Barbara Duden has contended that health as an individual's strife for medical well-being was not commonplace in the

7 While the early modern period is usually defined as beginning around 1450 in most of Europe, Swedish historians tend to locate the end of the Middle Ages to around 1500.

8 As exemplified in the recent special issues on the history of medicine in *Historisk Tidskrift* 143, no. 3 (2023) and *Historisk Tidskrift för Finland* 105, no. 4 (2020). For earlier studies with a wider chronological scope that situate meanings of health and illness in Swedish culture, see the works by Karin Johannisson, including *Medicinens öga* and *Kroppens tunna skal*.

9 Manning, 'Health in the Early Modern Philosophical Tradition,' 181.

early modern period.[10] The understanding of health in the early modern period was thus much broader and more diffused than the modern definition of health as bodily and mental well-being.[11] Studying health in this broad, early modern sense offers excellent opportunity to comprehend how people related their experiences of well-being or disease to daily practices, ideals, and the societies in which they lived.[12]

The social history of medicine has taken important steps in reading disease historically, paying attention to medical practice within as well as outside of medical institutions. However, previous scholarship has tended to focus its attention more on disease and illness, and less on contextualising health as a historical concept. Although David Harley had as early as 1999 pointed to the importance of studying health as socially constructed, less attention has been paid to the importance of historically contextualising the culturally embedded meaning and significance of 'health' than that of 'illness.'[13] Significant work has been undertaken in this regard in relation to the medieval period, but there is a need to take this discussion forward in time and to explore the understanding of health as a concept and a set of practices in the early modern period, as well as considering long-term change and continuity beyond the periodisations around which historians too often structure their analyses.[14]

When discussed in research, health as a concept is often seen in relation to disease or illness, and indeed, the etymological root of the words for health in Indo-European languages emphasise health as wholeness: health being the absence of injury, disease or illness.[15] That said, it is our contention that

10 Duden, *The Woman Beneath the Skin*, 16–19.

11 The World Health Organization constituted in 1946 that 'Health is a state of complete physical, mental and social well-being and not merely the absence of disease or infirmity.' See *World Health Organization*, 'Constitution.'

12 This focus highlights the quotidian practices and ideas of different people in various positions in society. Consequently, medical institutions and their impact on societal health form a backdrop rather than a focal point in this volume. For insights into the impact of various societal healthcare institutions in the early modern period in Sweden, see, e.g., Petersson, *Vadstena krigsmanshus*, Unger, *Makten och fattigdomen*, Blom, *Hospitalshjon och fribröder*, Blom, *Tiggare, tidstjuvar*. For an overview of early modern public healthcare in Norway and Denmark, see Moseng, *Ansvaret for undersåttenes helse.*

13 Harley, 'Rhetoric and the Social Construction of Sickness and Healing,' 420. Exceptions include Thomas, 'Health and Morality.'

14 On the medieval period, see essays in Ritchey and Strocchia, *Gender, Health, and Healing*. For an example of analysis stretching across traditional periodisation, see Foscati, *Saint Antony's Fire.*

15 Caplan, 'The Concepts of Health, Illness and Disease,' 239; Kontturi, 'Läkande, botande och bilden av den kompetenta medicinaren,' 503. On the etymology of health see Mallory and Adams, *Encyclopedia of Indo-European Culture*, 262.

health and illness should not be approached as having opposite meanings by default.

In philosophical discussions about the meaning of health, the early modern period has been pointed out as the moment in time when thinking about health changed into a matter of bodily well-being, largely following the French philosopher René Descartes, who emphasised a division between that which belongs to the body and that which belongs to the mind. It has been argued that the Cartesian division between mind and body led to the modern medical tradition, which focuses mainly on the well-being or disease of the body, while disregarding any effects the state of the body might have on the mind or spirit or vice versa, let alone the societal effects of bodily well-being or disease. Nevertheless, as Manning has pointed out, the early modern period was still firmly set in the ancient tradition, where the more holistic view of health described above was still influential.[16] Similarly, historians of the body and medicine have emphasised the degree to which mental states were understood to have bodily causes, and vice versa, in early modern society.[17] It seems, then, that the early modern period harboured both older and newer notions of health.

The confluence of older and newer conceptions of health is evident in the semantic variations of words used for health in the early modern period, and it can be exemplified through a survey of Swedish language use. The word for health in Swedish (Swe. *hälsa*) appeared in printed material in the early sixteenth century as a wish for the prosperity or welfare of a person. *The Swedish Academy Dictionary* (*SAOB*) notes a similar usage here to the Latin word 'salus.' Both terms were used as phrases of well-wishing that opened letters or other formalised statements. In this usage, the word *hälsa* referred to a person's prosperity or good fortune well beyond the medical sphere.[18]

At the same time, *hälsa* was used to refer more specifically to body and mind functioning in a satisfactory manner. For example, when, in 1527, King Gustavus Vasa granted an estate to 'his loyal subject' Olof Hattorsi, he noted that he expected Hattorsi to continue to show support 'as long as his health lasts.'[19] The king presumed that Hattorsi would be prepared to prove his loyalty as long as he was able. *SAOB* notes that from the seventeenth century, *hälsa* was used to refer in a related sense to the more general well-being of body and/or mind. It is significant that these usages were not altogether

16 Manning, 'Health in the Early Modern Philosophical Tradition,' 181–183.

17 Rublack, 'Fluxes'; Weisser, *Ill Composed*; Newton, 'Inside the Sickchamber.'

18 *SAOB*, 'hälsa subst.'

19 Gustavus Vasa, 'Förläningsbrev för Olof Hattorsi på hans fädernegård,' 125.

separate from health signifying prosperity. Indeed, in Stiernhielm's poem 'Hälse-Prijs,' health as the satisfactory state of body and mind is tied to the broader question of a person's prosperity.

Several words overlapped in meaning and usage with *hälsa*. One example of this is seen in the first Swedish translation of the Bible from 1541. The Book of Sirach 30:14 in the Swedish sixteenth-century version reads: 'It is better to be poor and to be healthy [Swe. *helbrägda*] and healthy [Swe. *frisk*], than rich and unhealthy [Swe. *osund*].'[20] Three words, near synonymous yet distinct, are used here to refer to health as a concept. The passage also expresses the sentiment we have already encountered in Stiernhielm's poem, namely that bodily and mental well-being is essential for a person's welfare, indicating the longer tradition that Stiernhielm was building on.

The first of the terms used to refer to health in the Book of Sirach is *helbrägda*. This word, uncommon today, was used in the early modern period primarily in the narrower sense of well-being in opposition to illness or injury, and sometimes as an adjective specifically denoting a contrast to a person or body part that was or had been unwell.[21] For instance, in a Swedish translation of the Icelandic historical epos *Heimskringla* from 1700, a character notes that 'I am still well [Swe. *helbrägd*] in my hands, yet weak in my feet.'[22] Here, the weakness of the feet is contrasted with the health of the hands.

SAOB also notes that *helbrägda* could be used to refer to a person who was 'unharmed.' This usage is seen in an anonymous account describing the reign of King Charles XII (1697–1718), written around the year 1750. In a passage that details the king's somewhat raucous evening entertainments, taking place when he was staying for a period in the southern Swedish town of Kristinehamn early in 1718, the reader is told that 'the ladies were happy when they escaped unharmed [*helbrägda*] from the game, and there was great perturbation about bruises on Princess Ulrica [Eleonora's] beautiful arms and hands.'[23] In this passage, *helbrägda* refers to the avoidance of harm, rather than a specific illness – a usage we will see recurring in several case studies in the present book. Moreover, while Charles XII's sister, later Queen Ulrica Eleonora (1719–1720), obtained bruises on her arms and hands, she is still described as having 'escaped unharmed.' How should we understand this comment? In this context, the term *helbrägda* more likely referred

20 *Biblia*, Syr 30:15. The Book of Sirach was translated into Swedish from the German Lutherbibel, and seems to have been popular in sixteenth century Sweden. Friesen, 'Inledning,' iii–ix.

21 *SAOB*, 'Helbrägda ssg'; 'Helbrägda sbst'; 'Helbrägda adj.'; 'Helbrägda v.'

22 Snorre Sturlason, *Heimskringla*, 2:202.

23 Anonymous, 'Facta till Revolutions-Historien,' 242.

to the ladies who had partaken in the games escaping with their virtue intact, rather than escaping bodily harm. Again, this is health as wholeness, though here referring to an intangible attribute – virtue – rather than to a bodily feature.

The association between health and virtue was expressed explicitly in Stiernhielm's monumental poem *Hercules*, where he asked: 'What is virtue, when virtue is the health [*hälsa*] of the soul?,' answering that 'virtue is loving ones God / to keep his commandment and laws.'[24] In this instance, Stiernhielm used the concept health metaphorically to express the sentiment that virtue is the essential good for the human soul, and from there connecting virtue to living life as a good Christian. In contrast, in the case of the carousing Princess Ulrica Eleonora and her accompanying noblewomen, the word *helbrägda* referred more concretely to the women's virtue being intact, rather than to health as a metaphor for a good outcome.

The adjective *sund* was used in opposition to ill health.[25] Indeed, we get an indication from this in the biblical passage Sirach 30:14, where *sund* is used with the preposition 'o-,' which has a negating meaning. In addition, however, both *sund*, *helbrägda*, and *hälsa* were used to refer to the quality of the surrounding environment, rather than to the human body.[26] Thus, the prominent civil servant Casten Feif commented to the architect Nicodemus Tessin about the streets of Stockholm that 'I find the air where I live much healthier [Swe. *sundare*] than up in the city among the narrow streets.'[27] The parts of the city Feif found healthy (Swe. *sunda*) were contrasted with those that were unhealthy (Swe. *osunda*), again delineating health as the opposite of ill health.

Of the three synonyms to the term *hälsa* that were used in the 1541 Bible translation, *frisk* was, and is, used with the most variation in meaning.[28] In early modern Swedish texts, *frisk*, related to English 'fresh,' could be used to describe something newly discovered or something unspoiled, as well as to refer to a person, item, or environment that was deemed to be in good condition. Similar to *sund*, *frisk* was used to refer to healthy air, as seen in a 1675 travel account that describes how the inhabitants of the city Carthagena in South America 'enjoy fresher [Swe. *friskare*] and healthier [Swe. *hälsosammare*] air, than those in surrounding locations.'[29] In this

24 Stiernhielm, *Hercules*, 36. This statement echoes conceptions of health and virtue in ancient philosophy. See Allen, 'The Soul's Virtue and the Health of the Body in Ancient Philosophy.'

25 *SAOB*, 'sund adj.'

26 See f.ex. *SAOB*, 'Helbrägda adj.'

27 Feif, 'Presidenten Frih. Casten Feifs Bref,' 147.

28 *SAOB*, 'frisk adj. 2.'

29 Anonymous, *Kort Berättelse om WästIndien*, 15.

passage, the word *frisk* is paired with health (Swe. *hälsosam* meaning 'being of good health'). Likewise, *frisk* was coupled with *sund*, as seen in the (now outdated) saying 'he is sound [*sund*] and fresh [*frisk*] like a fish,' used to describe a person who was particularly healthy.[30]

Similar to the usages sketched out above, *hälsa*, *helbrägda*, and *sund* – though not *frisk* – all had clear religious connotations. For example, the term *hälsa* was used as a metaphor to describe the nature of God as a saviour and his relationship to Christian believers as the salvation. Thus, Ephesians 5:23 in the first sixteenth-century Swedish translation of the New Testament reads, 'Christ is the head of the congregation, and he is the health of the body.'[31] Similarly, a sixteenth-century hymn declared that 'Jesus Christ is our health, who will save us all.'[32] In these examples, 'health' is a proxy for that which is good, to be compared with the same biblical passage in the King James Bible that uses 'saviour' in lieu of health. And indeed, Stiernhielm employed the word in its double religious meaning of saviour and salvation, when he described God as 'our eternal health' ('vår evige hälsa') at the end of the poem 'Hälse-Prijs.'[33]

In the references to Christ as the health of the congregation, we see a collective dimension of the concept of health. Here, health is not a question of the well-being of the individual, but rather, of the community. As Margaret Healy notes, society-wide illnesses such as the bubonic plague were often understood to have collective causes in early modern society and connected to failings of upholding Christian morals, while other illnesses were seen to have more individually attributable causes.[34] A collective aspect of 'health' is also noted in the realm of politics. Research on European political discourse and with regards to early modern Sweden has noted the use of health as a metaphor in politics, for example describing society as a body, or the king's body as a metaphor for society, and understanding political revolts as illnesses or dysfunctional limbs.[35]

30 Sparman, *Sundhetzens speghel*, 103.

31 *Thet nyia Testamentit på Swensko*, Ephesians 5:23. The same passage in King James version reads 'For the husband is the head of the wife, even as Christ is the head of the church: and he is the saviour of the body.'

32 [Olaus Petri]. 'Iesus Christus är wor helsa.' The psalm is Olaus Petri's Swedish translation of Luther's 'Jesus Christ, unser Heiland,' which in turn is a revision and expansion of the medieval hymn 'Jesus Christus, nostra salus.' We are grateful to Josef Eskhult for bringing our attention to this point.

33 Stiernhielm, 'Hälse-Prijs.'

34 Margaret Healy, 'Why Me? Why Now? How?'

35 Rönnqvist, *Der königliche Vater*, 141–155; Sennefelt, 'A Pathology'; Healy, *Fictions of Disease*. On the intersection between health, religion and kingship, see Brogan, *The Royal Touch in Early Modern England*.

A more comprehensive analysis of the meanings of health in the early modern period needs to pay attention, then, both to health as a concrete state of prosperity or the well-being of body and/or mind, and to health as a metaphor for good, often carrying political, moral, and religious overtones. Health was located in the individual person (in healthy hands but not in weak feet), in social relations (in the relation between two correspondents, and in the welfare of the political body or the Christian congregation), in the surrounding world (on the broad street more than on the narrow). Bearing this in mind, the tendency among scholars to problematise health to a lesser extent than illness, or simply use health as a contrasting state of being to illness, seems too limited for a comprehensive understanding of what health signified in the early modern period.

Moreover, when we probe the meaning of health, it is apparent that health is not necessarily a question primarily for medical practitioners, but an equally central matter in other areas of people's lives. None of the examples discussed in this short survey of the term come from medical practitioners or medical discourse, yet they were all part in conceptualising health in early modern society. It is our contention here that examining the historical meaning of health can be a way to further integrate the history of medicine into early modern history.

In this volume, the religious aspect of health is central in **Gabriela Bjarne Larsson**'s and **Riikka Miettinen**'s chapters. In her biographical study of a spice merchant turned Brigittine nun, Bjarne Larsson explores the complex relationship between parallel interpretative systems for understanding health at the end of the medieval period. Moving forward in time, Miettinen demonstrates how mental health was part of a religious discourse in rural communities in seventeenth- and early eighteenth-century Sweden. Through Miettinen's analysis, mental illness is revealed as something to be treated through religious guidance and ritual, the treatment often equally engaging kinship networks and local clergy. In both Miettinen and Bjarne Larsson's studies, religiously informed ideas and practices were central to how people conceived health, and the authors show how these ideas were intertwined with other knowledge regimes of healing.[36]

Another important paradigm for how people thought about health in early modern Sweden was the tradition of Galenic/Hippocratic medicine. The medical context in early modern Europe, in all its complexity, is highly influential as a conceptual framework for the analyses in this volume. In

36 On religion and medicine, see also Park, 'Medicine and Magic'; Grell and Cunningham, eds., *Medicine and the Reformation*; Grell and Cunningham, eds., *Medicine and Religion*.

the early modern period, scholarly inclined Europeans as well as the general populace largely adhered to the ideas of Galenic/Hippocratic medicine. In this tradition, a person was healthy when the four humours – blood, black bile, yellow bile, and phlegm – and their associated qualities were in balance in her body. Conversely, ill health resulted from an excess or lack of one or more of the humours. This theoretical framework led to therapies that aimed at adjusting a person's humoral balance, such as blood-letting, sweating, and purging. It also led to the widespread belief in preventive regimens governing daily activities like sleeping, eating, drinking, and exercising. These regimens emphasised moderation in all things, with the belief that this would help preserve a beneficial humoral balance. From the perspective of Galenic medicine, a healthy body was a body in balance.

This paradigm of thought remained influential throughout the seventeenth and well into the eighteenth century in Sweden, and some ideas and practices continued to be important at an even later date. For example, the abandonment of miasmatic medicine and climate theory – both important elements of Galenic/Hippocratic medicine – has been located to the mid-nineteenth century in Sweden.[37]

At the same time, the early modern period also saw the introduction of new medical paradigms for understanding health.[38] One such system was the chemically informed view of the Paracelsian iatrochemists, who understood sulphur, mercury, and salt, rather than the humours, to be essential to medicine. This understanding resulted in an increased influence of chemical remedies in learned medicine.[39] Another important viewpoint was the iatromechanic understanding of medicine, in which the body was thought of as a functioning or dysfunctioning machine.[40]

These medical theories continually influenced each other in the learned debate of the period and were often combined in pragmatic ways.[41] Several of the chapters in this volume offer insights into how these theories were discussed and applied in various contexts. The iatromechanic understanding of medicine is usually portrayed as a theoretically informed standpoint, yet in his contribution to this volume, **Anton Runesson** shows how similar ideas about health and illness were held among the broader populace in early

37 Drakman, *När kroppen slöt sig och blev fast*, 19.

38 Murphy provides a view of what this could mean for an individual practitioner, see Murphy, 'Common Places and Private Spaces.'

39 On Paracelsian ideas in Sweden, see Karlsson, *Götisk kabbala och runisk alkemi*, 95–97; Lindroth, *Paracelsismen*, for influence on medicine, especially 447–468.

40 Dunér, 'Maskinen människa.'

41 Gentilcore, *Food and Health in Early Modern Europe*, 35–36.

modern Sweden.[42] Rather than seeing this as a top-down spread of certain ideas, Runesson shows how the notion of health related to the importance of being able to work in the local community. Moreover, by exploring how the reading difficulties of the Swedish King Charles XI were dealt with, **Andreas Hellerstedt** highlights a pragmatic approach to Galenic theory: the young king's teacher mitigated the fact that Charles XI lacked certain talents expected from a king by renegotiating the theory of the temperaments. By analysing the case of Charles XI, Hellerstedt highlights how the meaning of health had importance in early modern politics and pedagogy.

The significance of social relations located in specific places of healing is further highlighted in **Charlotta Forss**'s study of the sauna as a place people visited when they felt unwell. She shows how people considered the act of using the bathhouse, or sauna, as a means of preserving or restoring health. This embedded notions of health in everyday life, since sweat baths were also a widespread social pastime in early modern Sweden and Finland. Moreover, **Maria Sjöberg** and **Hedvig Widmalm** give examples of how health was tied to gendered social relations. Widmalm makes an important point in highlighting how the conceptual associations between hair and health changed over time, and that gender was a crucial component for these changes. While several contributions of the volume highlight the importance of holistic ideas of health in the period, Widmalm's study shows how the conception of health could equally be tied to a particular body part. Sjöberg instead approaches early modern understandings of health through examining the changing nature of the medical marketplace. In so doing, she highlights the centrality of gendered ideas of work in the way healthcare professions emerged.

In his revisionist account of the role and status of Swedish physicians in the eighteenth century, **Hjalmar Fors** probes our conceptions of the early modern medical marketplace from a different perspective. He shows how social relations beyond the medical sphere were central for practitioners, for example in the networks of patrons that physicians drew on, and in the way the state related to physicians as one among many groups of civil servants. This view is a reminder that health practices did not circulate in a closed-off sphere. Quite the contrary: notions of health were conceptualised in relation to myriad relations, practices, and institutions that filled people's lives.

Together, the contributions in this volume offer rich insights into the different social contexts in which the meanings of health were shaped in

42 In a study of post-partum narratives in early modern England, Lea Astbury similarly emphasises the importance of the functionality of the body in daily life for early modern conceptions of health. See Astbury, 'Being Well, Looking Ill.'

early modern Sweden. They testify to the multitude of traditions, norms, and ideas that informed the understanding of health and to the diverse set of practices that aimed at maintaining or improving it. They show how the notion of health was omnipresent in early modern society and made up a framework for living a good life.

Health and healthcare in early modern Sweden

In this section, we outline some important features of early modern Swedish society in relation to health and healthcare, and situate the chapters of the volume within this framework. Late medieval and early modern Sweden, including present-day Finland, constitutes the chronological and geographical framework of this volume. The sixteenth century, where the volume begins, saw Sweden emerge as a fledgling independent state. During the next two hundred years, Sweden grew in terms of territory as well as in terms of its military and political ambitions. At the height of influence, in the second half of the seventeenth century, Sweden was a Baltic superpower, and the country was deeply involved in the struggles for dominance on the continent. The dawn of the eighteenth century saw a reversal of fortunes in the Great Northern War (1700–1721), and by necessity, Sweden took on a less expansionist role in the following century.[43]

These political developments make for a dramatic backdrop to our set of chapters. For some – like Andreas Hellerstedt's study of the reading difficulties of King Charles XI – the political framework is highly relevant for interpreting how notions of health were understood and used. In other contributions, processes such as religious life after the Reformation – in Riikka Miettinen's chapter – or changing consumer patterns in the late eighteenth and early nineteenth centuries – in Hedvig Widmalm's – are of greater import. For all authors, contextual readings have proven crucial for understanding the developments they study.

That said, while the focus of the volume is on Sweden, the historical understanding of health is in no way solely dependent on a national context but rather emerges through a network of influences.[44] Throughout the early modern period, Sweden was closely connected to surrounding areas in terms

43 See further Lindkvist, Sjöberg, Hedenborg, and Kvarnström, *A Concise History of Sweden*; Villstrand, *Sveriges Historia*; Lockhart, *Sweden in the Seventeenth Century*.

44 On the importance of cross-cultural transmissions for the history of medicine, see Alberts, Fransen, and Leong, eds., *Translating Medicine across Premodern Worlds*.

of movement of peoples and ideas. For example, though it was possible to study medicine at Swedish institutions of learning in the early modern period, many students conducted part of their studies abroad, at German, Dutch, and, in the eighteenth century, French universities. A doctorate degree in medicine was offered in Sweden only from 1737.[45] When it came to scholarly literature on medicine and medical advice books (Swe. *läke- och örteböcker*) aimed at a broader audience, most medieval Swedish volumes were translations of German and Danish works. Well into the seventeenth century, much of the Swedish-language advice literature on healing drew on German and French publications.[46]

Still, the books written with a Swedish audience in mind were not simply translations. Indicating the local adaptations and the significance given to local conditions by historical actors, the present volume brings an often-overlooked perspective on ideas and practices of healing in Northern Europe to the discussion of early modern European health. For instance, Charlotta Forss considers how early modern Swedish medical authors argued that they adjusted their advice to local contexts, so that it would be efficiently useful for people 'in these Northerly lands.' In contrast, Widmalm highlights how eighteenth-century Swedish critics of wig-wearing worried that the new fashion had *not* been localised and thus would endanger health. Together, these chapters capture how historical actors themselves made use of a localised understanding of health to promote their own agenda.

This attention to how the understanding of health was localised is a valuable contribution to a broader discussion about health in early modern Europe. To begin with, the case studies in this volume provide points of comparison with developments elsewhere, thus nuancing and enriching our understanding of what health was and could be in different societal contexts. Moreover, the chapters draw attention to the analytical potential of focusing on how knowledge about the human body was made and legitimated. We see time and again how social practices – like working or bathing – were central to how early modern people conceptualised health itself. The history of knowledge has pointed to the importance of looking at processes through which knowledge was made and vocalised.[47] This volume

45 Maaniitty, 'Befolknings- och folkhälsofrågornas framväxt,' 443; See also Hult, 'Frankriket i svensk medicin.'

46 Christenson Nugues, 'Skolmedicinen i det medeltida Sverige,' 71; With regards to almanacs (a genre which often included medical advice), see Nordenmark, *Naturvetenskapernas historia i Sverige*, 73.

47 See, e.g., Daston, 'The History of Science'; Lässing, 'The History of Knowledge.' For the history of knowledge in Scandinavian historical research, see Östling et al., 'The History of Knowledge.'

provides case studies of how this tenet can be set into practical use within the field of health and illness.

The importance of studying health beyond present-day geographical borders can also be seen when considering networks of people and institutions. In a biographical study that problematises the methodological nationalism inherent in a study of health and society in early modern Sweden, Gabriela Bjarne Larsson takes the example of Maihingen in Southern Germany. Bjarne Larsson demonstrates that the institutional framework of the Brigittine order, with its central node in Swedish Vadstena, was as important a reference point for the healing practices that were carried out at the convent as the local culture in Maihingen. She shows how different knowledge regimes for interpreting health and combating illness were combined through the personal experiences and resources of individuals entering the Brigittine convent. At the same time, she makes clear that the religious institution, the Brigittine monastery, created a framework for interpreting health in the period.

Bjarne Larsson's study is set at the cusp of the early modern period, in the early sixteenth century. In the following decades, the Reformation restructured private devotion and the institutions for healing in Sweden and much of Europe.[48] Religious houses and monasteries in the Swedish realm, as well as the houses of healing tied to monasteries (Swe. *helgeandshus*), were closed in the wake of the Reformation. Secular institutions that provided care, so called *hospitals*, became more important in cities and towns.[49] The defining factors for receiving care at a hospital were, first, whether a person was in need of help for their survival, and, second, if they followed the rules of proper behaviour set out by the institution. As noted by earlier research, this meant that the old, the very young, the disabled, and those suffering from severe illnesses were grouped together conceptually and institutionally.[50]

There were a number of different persons, places, and institutions that people in early modern Sweden turned to when looking for the treatment of bodily or mental symptoms of ill-health. In Stockholm and the larger towns of the realm, several groups of medical practitioners complemented and competed with each other.[51] One group of healthcare practitioners which has

48 Grell and Cunningham, 'The Reformation and Changes in Welfare Provision,' 1–41.

49 Broberg, 'Liten svensk medicinhistoria,' 14.

50 Sandén, 'I livets skuggdalar,' 49–72; Nordström, *Vården och staten*, 45.

51 On early modern Swedish medical professions, see, e.g., Lindberg, *Peregrinatio medica*; Lindberg, *Kirurgernas historia*; Vainio-Korhonen, *De frimodiga*; Fors, 'Medicine and the Making of a City'; Bergqvist, *Läkare och läkande*.

received plenty of attention, but whose roles at the early modern medical marketplace still remain a point of contention, are university trained physicians. In Sweden, the 1663 founding of the Collegium Medicum, which had oversight duties for other medical professions for most of the early modern period, has traditionally been seen as an important point in the gradual professionalisation of physicians as the foremost providers of care.[52] Hjalmar Fors's chapter makes an important contribution to this debate by not only situating the physicians in relation to other healthcare practitioners, but also comparing their roles to other groups of actors associated with the state bureaucracy, which, from the seventeenth century, grew in scope as well as personnel. Viewed in this light, the role of the Swedish physicians in the eighteenth century appears much less exceptional. Physicians comprised one group among many who performed functions in the state. Compared to other groups, such as the civil servants of the Bureau of Mines (Swe. *Bergskollegium*), the mandates and status of the physicians appear unimpressive.

These insights are interesting not least in relation to the broader account of early modern medical history. Earlier research has noted that, with regards to institutional developments in healthcare, early modern Sweden appears to have been somewhat behind general European trends. This is not least because medical professionalisation developed there later than in many other parts of Europe.[53] This circumstance constitutes another argument for including the early modern period in its widest possible sense, as is done in this volume.

Another way to contextualise early modern medical practitioners is to consider how their practice was structured in relation to important forces at work in society at large. In a close examination of how gender norms shaped the medical marketplace, Maria Sjöberg points to the household as an important institution for healthcare practitioners at the beginning of the early modern period, arguing that 'a barber's activity was perceived as based on marriage and family.' As such, women most likely figured as healthcare providers to a greater degree than the formal, and male-coded, regulations indicate. Sjöberg traces the history of the barber-surgeons up to around 1900, a move that allows her to map out long-term changes in the gender coding of the work of the barber-surgeons. She observes that while women were allowed to formally train to become barber-surgeons in the nineteenth century, this coincided with the occupation's loss of status. Her

52 See Hjelt, *Svenska och finska medicinalverkets historia*, 1:3; Wolff, 'Kirurgerna och förnyelsen av läkarvetenskapen,' 470–496; Stolberg, 'Learning from the Common Folks,' 649–667.
53 Bergqvist, *Läkare och läkande*.

chapter highlights the significance of regulation, both in creating a space for female healthcare practitioners and also, paradoxically, in setting the stage for control and curtailing the activities of women. Taken together, Hjalmar Fors and Maria Sjöberg's chapters provide a more historically sensitive reading of the role and status of early modern medical practitioners.

Focusing on the place rather than the performers of healing, Charlotta Forss's chapter examines the role of the sweat bath, or sauna, in early modern Sweden. Her analysis highlights that visiting the sauna was a way to enact health or illness. Expressing the wish to take a bath could be used as evidence of illness, but the actual bath was also considered to treat a number of ailments and to prevent a person from falling ill. With this perspective, Forss brings much-needed attention to one of the places where people sought healing in early modern society. In the bathhouse, a person feeling unwell could receive advice and treatments from trained physicians, barbers, or bathers, but equally, they could be treated by a person in the local community who was considered to be knowledgeable in healing, or they could be helped by friends or family, or, indeed, engage in self-care. Focusing on the places where healing was conducted helps bring new depth to the well-established fact that early modern people drew on health advice from several different groups of actors and knowledge regimes. In addition, Forss's perspective emphasises a situational understanding of health through highlighting how health was defined both in relation to the bathhouse as a place, and in relation to the characteristics of the bodies who frequented the bath.

In their respective chapters, Riikka Miettinen and Anton Runesson challenge the bias of giving interpretative primacy to the urban environment over the rural setting found in earlier research. The countryside was, after all, the arena where most people in early modern Sweden lived out their lives. Indeed, earlier research has noted that, with regards to Sweden, studies of rural conditions and of everyday practices of medicine have to date been only partial.[54] Both authors make use of court records, as does Charlotta Forss in her study of health in the bathhouse, as a means to gain insight into health practices beyond the learned elite. Miettinen's chapter deals with responses to mental illness in rural communities during the seventeenth and eighteenth centuries. Through her analysis, it becomes apparent that notions of health and well-being were deeply immersed in communal life. The health or ill-health of members of the community was a matter of importance for family and friends. Moreover, the clergy seems to have taken an active role in supporting those who suffered, as

54 Drakman, *När kroppen slöt sig*, 23, 36.

well as administering treatments that were understood to have a healing or alleviating potential. These treatments could consist of prayers or the administration of sacraments.

Runesson focuses less on healing activities and more on how people in rural communities spoke about bodily health. Specifically, he makes use of witness testimonies in court protocols to tease out the conceptualisation of illness among a stratum of the population who are not normally heard. Runesson emphasises the importance of recognising that rural communities understood illness as a lack of ability to perform one's usual tasks. Bodily ailments were related to a person's position in the local community and to the importance of providing sustenance, rather than to humoral conceptions of the causes and effects of disease or injury. Here, we see a parallel to the function of an early modern Swedish hospital, which, literally and symbolically, brought people who could not provide for themselves together under one roof.

Not all symptoms that are today regarded as part of the medical sphere were considered as such in early modern worldviews, although they were informed by humoral thinking about the human constitution. In his chapter, Andreas Hellerstedt argues that the learning difficulties of King Charles XI were *not* considered a question of health. Rather, the young king's teacher, Edmund Gripenhielm, interpreted Charles's reading difficulties as a natural variation of temperament. In part, this conclusion could be reached through reasoning about the variance of the composition of the four humours which gave every person their individual character. Despite the young king's inability to succeed in the ambitious education commensurate with a monarch's role, the political impossibility of declaring the king mentally slow or stupid was evident and shaped Gripenhielm's reasoning about the four humours. Gripenhielm needed to come to the conclusion that the king was too talented, rather than not talented enough or lacking in some area. Hellerstedt demonstrates how this political reality influenced the interpretation of medical theory.

In the eighteenth century, a growing priority of the state to manage its population was paired with new scientific ideals and interests in investigating the human body and mind. These combined forces led to, among other things, the founding of new institutions to investigate, educate, and manage health. Of particular concern to the eighteenth-century Swedish elite was the fact that the country was so sparsely populated.[55] *Serafimerlasarettet*, a teaching hospital, was founded in 1752, and attempts were made to gather

55 Maaniitty, 'Befolknings- och folkhälsofrågornas framväxt,' 441–469.

information about the health of the population through yearly reports from physicians and from parishes.[56] Carolus Linnaeus, in addition to his classifications of plants, animals and humans, provided classifications of illnesses.[57]

Consumer patterns shifted and evolved in the eighteenth and nineteenth centuries. One area where this is evident is hair fashion, and in her chapter, Hedvig Widmalm takes us through the fascinating elements of thought and practice in how people in Sweden related to their hair in the period 1740 to 1840. She shows how wigs – primarily worn by men of the elite in Sweden – were considered a dangerous and potentially unhealthy influence by critics in the late eighteenth century. In contrast, an emerging genre of cosmetic advice books in the nineteenth century emphasised the connection between, on the one hand, female hairstyles, and, on the other, ideals of beauty and attractiveness. Consequently, with regards to hair, health became a question of gender. Widmalm demonstrates how this gendering of health through hair came about through changing fashion trends and consumer patterns. Focusing on hair also allows her to highlight the porous borders between questions of health, food, beauty, and ideas about good householding in the early modern period, as advice books tended to treat these topics in tandem.

Taken together, the chapters that make up this volume bring attention to an array of societal factors that were instrumental for shaping early modern medical practice. And conversely, the contributors show how ideas and practices that have been related primarily to medical history had an import well beyond that sphere. The classical narrative in European history of early medicine and health is broadened and at times challenged by the focus on Sweden. Institutional developments occurred at a different pace in the northern peripheries of Europe, and the specific societal context influenced the formation of medical professions as well as the conceptual framework of how health was understood.

Finally, the question raised in the beginning of this introduction – what is health? – has a bearing far beyond the early modern period. In her concluding epilogue, **Helena Tolvhed** uses the early modern conceptions of health outlined in the chapters of this volume as a starting point for reflecting about the meaning of health in the twentieth and twenty-first centuries. She shows how the holistic understanding of health that was prominent in the early modern period has much in common with the

56 Broberg, 'Liten svensk medicinhistoria,' 17–19.
57 Broberg, 'Liten svensk medicinhistoria,' 17–18.

present-day discourse. Equally important, Tolvhed reveals how societal change continuously redefines the relations between health and society, even to this day.

Bibliography

Printed works

Anonymous. 'Facta till Revolutions-Historien under Konung Carl XIIs Regering, Drottning Ulrica Eleonoras samt början af Konung Fredrics; med teckning af diverse dihörande personers lynnen.' In *Handlingar rörande Skandinaviens Historia*, vol. 7. Stockholm: Elmeéns och Granbergs Tryckeri, 1819.

Anonymous. *Kort Berättelse om WästIndien eller America, som elliest kallas Nya Werlden*, edited by Johann Kankel. Visingsö, 1675.

[Olaus Petri]. 'Iesus Christus är wor helsa.' In *Swenske songer eller wisor nw på nytt prentade, förökade, och vnder en annan skick än tilförenna vtsatte*. Stockholm, 1536.

Biblia / Thet är / All then Helgha Scrifft / på Swensko [*Gustavus Vasa's bibel*]. Uppsala, 1541.

Feif, Casten. 'Presidenten Frih. Casten Feifs Bref till Kongl. Rådet Gr. Nicodemus Tessin.' In *Handlingar ur v. Brinkmanska archivet på Trolle-Ljungby*, edited by Gustav Andersson, vol. 1, 143–149. Örebro, 1859.

Gustavus Vasa,'Förläningsbrev för Olof Hattorsi på hans fädernegård.' In *Konung Gustaf den förstes registratur*, vol. IV. Stockholm: P.A. Norstedt & söner, 1868.

Holy Bible: King James Version. Cambridge: Cambridge University Press, 2017.

Snorre Sturlason. *Heims Kringlans eller Snorre Sturlusons andra band, innehållandes historierna om konung Magnus the gode, och the följande norländska konungar. = Sive Historiarum regum septentrionalium tomus secundus, continens res præcipue gestas Magni ... Ex Sturlonidœ contextu antiquo, versione gemina illustratus a Johanne Peringskiold*. Translated by Johan Peringskiöld. [Stockholm, 1700.]

Stiernhielm, Georg. *Hercules*. Uppsala, 1658.

Stiernhielm, Georg. 'Hälse-Prijs.' In *Musas Suethizantes Thet är Sång-Gudinnor, Nu först lärande Dichta och Spela på Swenska*. Stockholm, 1668.

Sparman, Andreas. *Sundhetzens speghel, vthi hwilken man beskodhar sundhetzens natur, förnämste orsakerne til alla siukdomar, som sundheten förstöra plägha, såsom ock the medels rätta brwk, hwarigenom hon för them befrijat, til thet bestämda målet kan underhållen warda*. Stockholm, 1642.

Thet nyia Testamentit på Swensko af år 1526. Published by Aksel Andersson. Uppsala: Akademiska boktryckeriet, 1893.

Literature

Alberts, Tara, Sietske Fransen, and Elaine Leong, eds. 'Translating Medicine across Premodern Worlds.' Special issue, *Osiris* 37 (2022).

Allen, James. 'The Soul's Virtue and the Health of the Body in Ancient Philosophy.' In *Health: A History*, edited by Peter Adamson, 180–221. Oxford: Oxford University Press, 2019.

Annola, Johanna, Annelie Drakman, and Marie Ulväng, eds. *Med tvål, vatten och flit: Hälsofrämjande renlighet som ideal och praktik ca 1870–1930*. Lund: Nordic Academic Press, 2021.

Astbury, Lea. 'Being Well, Looking Ill: Childbirth and the Return to Health in Seventeenth-Century England.' *Social History of Medicine* 30, no. 3 (2017): 500–519.

Bergqvist, Johanna. *Läkare och läkande: Läkekonstens professionalisering i Sverige under medeltid och renässans*. Lund: Lund Studies in Historical Archaeology, 2013.

Blom, Conny. *Hospitalshjon och fribröder: de äldres villkor inom den offentliga vården från senmedeltiden till 1700-talets slut*. Uppsala: Sociologiska institutionen, Uppsala universitet, 1991.

Blom, Conny. *Tiggare, tidstjuvar, lättingar och landstrykare: studier av attityder och värderingar i skrån, stadgar, ordningar och lagförslag gällande den offentliga vården 1533–1664*. Lund: Lund University Press, 1992.

Broberg, Gunnar. 'Liten svensk medicinhistoria.' In *Til at stwdera läkedom: Tio studier i svensk medicinhistoria*, edited by Gunnar Broberg, 9–50. Lund: Sekel, 2008.

Brogan, Stephen. *The Royal Touch in Early Modern England. Politics, Medicine and Sin*. Woodbridge: Boydell Press, 2015.

Caplan, Arthur L., 'The Concepts of Health, Illness and Disease.' In *Companion Encyclopedia of the History of Medicine*, edited by W.F. Bynum and Roy Porter, 233–248. London: Routledge, 1993.

Carrera, Elena, ed. *Emotions and Health, 1200–1700*. Leiden: Brill, 2013.

Christenson Nugues, Charlotte. 'Skolmedicinen i det medeltida Sverige: En historia från Europas periferi.' In *Til at stwdera läkedom: Tio studier i svensk medicinhistoria*, edited by Gunnar Broberg, 61–77. Lund: Sekel, 2008.

Daston, Lorraine. 'The History of Science and the History of Knowledge.' *KNOW: A Journal on the Formation of Knowledge* 1, no. 1 (2017): 131–154.

Drakman, Annelie. *När kroppen slöt sig och blev fast: Varför åderlåtning, miasmateori och klimatmedicin övergavs vid 1800-talets mitt*. Uppsala: Acta Universitatis Upsaliensis, 2018.

Duden, Barbara. *The Woman beneath the Skin: A Doctor's Patients in Eighteenth-Century Germany*. Cambridge, MA: Harvard University Press, 1991.

Dunér, David. 'Maskinen människa.' In *Til at stwdera läkedom: Tio studier i svensk medicinhistoria*, edited by Gunnar Broberg, 111–149. Lund: Sekel, 2008.

Fors, Hjalmar. 'Medicine and the Making of a City: Spaces of Pharmacy and Scholarly Medicine in Seventeenth-Century Sweden.' *Isis* 107, no. 3 (2016): 473–494.

Foscati, Alessandra. *Saint Antony's Fire from Antiquity to the Eighteenth Century*. Amsterdam: Amsterdam University Press, 2019.

Friesen, Otto von. 'Inledning.' In *Jesu Syrachs bok I 1541 års svenska bibel*, edited by Otto von Friesen, iii–xxxviii, Uppsala: Akademiska bokhandeln, 1912.

Gentilcore, David. *Food and Health in Early Modern Europe: Diet, Medicine and Society, 1450–1800*. London: Bloomsbury Academic, 2015.

Grell, Ole Peter, and Andrew Cunningham, eds. *Medicine and the Reformation*. London and New York: Routledge, 1993.

Grell, Ole Peter, and Andrew Cunningham, eds. *Medicine and Religion in Enlightenment Europe*. Aldershot: Ashgate, 2006.

Grell, Ole Peter, and Andrew Cunningham. 'The Reformation and Changes in Welfare Provision.' In *Health Care and Poor Relief in Protestant Europe 1500–1700*, edited by Ole Peter Grell and Andrew Cunningham, 1–41. London: Routledge, 1997.

Harley, David. 'Rhetoric and the Social Construction of Sickness and Healing.' *Social History of Medicine* vol. 12, no. 3 (1999), 407–435.

Healy, Margaret. *Fictions of Disease in Early Modern England: Bodies, Plagues and Politics*. New York: Palgrave, 2001.

Healy, Margaret. 'Why Me? Why Now? How? The Body in Health and Disease.' In *A Cultural History of the Human Body in the Renaissance*, edited by Linda Kalof and W. F. Bynum, 37–54. Oxford: Berg Publishers, 2010.

Historisk Tidskrift 143, no. 3 (2023).

Historisk Tidskrift för Finland 105, no. 4 (2020).

Hjelt, Otto E. A. *Svenska och finska medicinalverkets historia 1663–1812*, vol. 1. Helsinki: Helsingfors centraltryckeri, 1891.

Hult, O.T. 'Frankriket i svensk medicin under 16- och 1700-talen.' *Lychnos* (1940): 274–299.

Johannisson, Karin. *Kroppens tunna skal: Sex essäer om kropp, historia och kultur*. Stockholm: Norstedts, 2013.

Johannisson, Karin. *Medicinens öga: Sjukdom, medicin och samhälle – historiska erfarenheter*. Stockholm: Norstedts, 2013.

Kalof, Linda, and W. F. Bynum, eds. *A Cultural History of the Human Body in the Renaissance*. Oxford: Berg Publishers, 2010.

Karlsson, Thomas. *Götisk kabbala och runisk alkemi: Johannes Bureus och den götiska esoterismen*. Stockholm: Stockholms universitet, 2010.

Kontturi, Saara-Maija. 'Läkande, botande och bilden av den kompetenta medicinaren i de finländska läkarnas årsberättelser 1769–1856.' *Historisk Tidskrift för Finland* 105, no. 4 (2020), 497–515.

Koselleck, Reinhart. *The Practice of Conceptual History: Timing History, Spacing Concepts.* Stanford, CA: Stanford University Press, 2002.

Lindberg, Bo S. *Kirurgernas historia: Om badare, barberare och fältskärer.* Uppsala: Uppsala University, 2017.

Lindberg, Bo S. *Peregrination medica: Svenska medicinares studieresor i Europa 1600–1800.* Uppsala: Uppsala University, 2019.

Lindemann, Mary. *Medicine and Society in Early Modern Europe.* Cambridge: Cambridge University Press, 2010.

Lindkvist, Thomas, Maria Sjöberg, Susanna Hedenborg, and Lars Kvarnström. *A Concise History of Sweden from the Viking Age to the Present.* Lund: Studentlitteratur, 2018.

Lindroth, Sten. *Paracelsismen i Sverige till 1600-talets mitt.* Uppsala and Stockholm: Almqvist & Wiksell, 1943.

Ling, Sofia. *Kärringmedicin och vetenskap: Läkare och kvacksalverianklagade i Sverige omkring 1770–1870.* Uppsala: Acta Universitatis Upsaliensis, 2004.

Lockhart, Paul Douglas. *Sweden in the Seventeenth Century.* Basingstoke: Palgrave Macmillan, 2004.

Lässing, Simone. 'The history of knowledge and the expansion of the Historical Research Agenda.' *Bulletin of the German Historical Institute* 59 (2016): 29–58.

Maaniitty, Elina. 'Befolknings- och folkhälsofrågornas framväxt och läkarnas förändrade yrkesbild i Sverige på 1700-talet.' *Historisk tidskrift för Finland* 105, no. 4 (2020): 441–469.

Mallory, J. P., and Douglas Q. Adams. *Encyclopedia of Indo-European Culture.* London and Chicago: Fitzroy Dearborn, 1997.

Manning, Gideon. 'Health in the Early Modern Philosophical Tradition.' In *Health: A History,* edited by Peter Adamson, 180–221. Oxford: Oxford University Press, 2019.

Moseng, Ole Georg. *Ansvaret for undersåttenes helse 1603–1850.* Oslo: Universitetsforlaget, 2003.

Murphy, Hannah. 'Common Places and Private Spaces: Libraries, Record-Keeping and Orders of Information in Sixteenth-Century Medicine.' *Past and Present Supplement* 11 (2016): 253–268.

Newton, Hannah. 'Inside the Sickchamber in Early Modern England: The Experience of Illness through Six Objects.' *English Historical Review* 136, no. 580 (2021): 530–567.

Nilsson, Anna. *Lyckans betydelse. Sekularisering, sensibilisering och individualisering i svenska skillingtryck 1750–1850.* Höör: Agering, 2012.

Nordenmark, N. V. E. *Naturvetenskapernas historia i Sverige intill år 1800, del 2: Astronomiens historia i Sverige till år 1800.* Uppsala: Almqvist & Wiksell, 1959.

Nordström, Åke. *Vården och staten: Källor till hälso- och sjukvårdens historia från medeltiden till 1967*, vol. 1. Stockholm: Skrifter utgivna av Riksarkivet 41, 2020.

North, Susan. *Sweet and Clean? Bodies and Clothes in Early Modern England.* Oxford: Oxford University Press, 2020.

Olsson, Bernt. 'Georg Stiernhielm.' *Svenskt biografiskt lexikon.* https://sok.riksarkivet.se/sbl/Presentation.aspx?id=20162. Accessed 1 September 2022.

Östling, Johan, David Larsson Heidenblad, Erling Sandmo, Anna Nilsson Hammar, and Kari Nordberg. 'The History of Knowledge and the Circulation of Knowledge: An Introduction.' In *Circulation of Knowledge: Explorations into the History of Knowledge*, edited by Johan Östling, Erling Sandmo, David Larsson Heidenblad, Anna Nilsson Hammar, and Kari Nordberg. Lund: Nordic Academic Press, 2018.

Park, Katherine. 'Medicine and Magic: The Healing Arts.' In *Gender and Society in Renaissance Italy*, edited by Judith C. Brown and Robert C. Davis, 129–149. London: Routledge, 1998.

Petersson, Erik. *Vadstena krigsmanshus: en studie av den svenska kronans inrättning för sårade och gamla soldater cirka 1640–1780.* Linköping: Institutionen för studier av samhällsutveckling och kultur, Linköpings universitet, 2017.

Porter, Roy. 'The Patient's View: Doing Medical History from Below.' *Theory and Society* 14, no. 2 (1985): 175–198.

Ritchey, Sara Margaret, and Sharon T. Strocchia, eds. *Gender, Health, and Healing, 1250–1550.* Amsterdam: Amsterdam University Press, 2020.

Rublack, Ulinka. 'Fluxes: The Early Modern Body and the Emotions.' *History Workshop Journal* 53 (2002): 1–16.

Rönnqvist, Miriam. *Der königliche Vater und seine ungehorsamen Kinder Furcht vor Bauernrevolten, Revoltenkommunikation und politische Kultur im frühneuzeitlichen schwedischen Reich.* Åbo: Åbo Akademis förlag, 2022.

Sandén, Annika. 'I livets skuggdalar, Fattigdom och överlevnad i reformationstidens Sverige.' In *Usla, eländа och arma: Samhällets utsatta under 700 år*, edited by Sofia Holmlund and Annika Sandén, 49–72. Stockholm: Natur och kultur, 2013.

Savin, Kristiina. *Fortunas klädnader: Lycka olycka och risk i det tidigmoderna Sverige.* Lund: Sekel, 2011.

Sennefelt, Karin. 'A Pathology of Sacred Kingship: Putrefaction in the Body of Charles XI of Sweden.' *Past & Present* 253 (2021): 83–117.

Smith, Virginia. *Clean: A History of Personal Hygiene and Purity.* Oxford: Oxford University Press, 2007.

Stolberg, Michael. 'Learning from the Common Folks: Academic Physicians and Medical Lay Culture in the Sixteenth Century.' *Social History of Medicine* 27, no. 4 (2014): 649–667.

Swedish Academy Dictionary (*SAOB*). Online: https://www.saob.se/in-english/.
Thomas, Keith. 'Health and Morality in Early Modern England.' In *Morality and Health*, edited by Allan M. Brandt and Paul Rozin, 15–34. New York: Routledge, 1997.
Unger, Christina. *Makten och fattigdomen: Fattigpolitik och fattigvård i 1600-talets Stockholm*. Stockholm: Stockholmia, 1996.
Vainio-Korhonen. *De Frimodiga: Barnmorskor, födande och kroppslighet på 1700-talet*. Helsinki: Svenska Literatursällskapet i Finland, 2016.
Van Bavel, Bas. 'The Economic Origins of Cleanliness in the Dutch Golden Age.' *Past & Present* 205 (2009): 41–69.
Villstrand, Nils Erik. *Sveriges Historia: 1600–1721*. Stockholm: Norstedts förlag, 2011.
Weisser, Olivia. *Ill Composed: Sickness, Gender and Belief in Early Modern England*. New Haven, CT and London: Yale University Press, 2016.
Williams, Raymond. *Keywords: A Vocabulary of Culture and Society*. New York: Oxford University Press, [1976] 1983.
Wolff, Charlotta. 'Kirurgerna och förnyelsen av läkarvetenskapen i Finland 1751–1850.' *Historisk Tidskrift för Finland* 105, no. 4 (2020): 470–496.
World Health Organization, 'Constitution.' https://www.who.int/about/governance/constitution. Accessed 1 September 2022.

About the authors

Charlotta Forss is an Associate Senior Lecturer, Department of Historical and Contemporary Studies, Södertörn University. Her current research examines how notions of health and morality were renegotiated in the early modern bathhouse culture of Sweden and Finland. Her upcoming book, Mapping the idea of North (Oxford: Bodleian Publishing, 2025) explores the connection between conceptions of climate and people on maps.

Mari Eyice is a Researcher at the Department of History, Stockholm University. In her current research, she explores how emotional practices were shaped in relation to disability in the early modern period. Her publications include 'Experiencing the dis/abled body in Early Modern Sweden: an exploration of perspectives' (*Memini: Travaux et Documents*, vol. 28, 2022.

2. Illness as Incapacity to Work in Early Modern Sweden

Anton Runesson

Abstract
The chapter analyses the meanings of 'illness' and 'incapacity' in early modern Swedish criminal investigations. In so doing, it challenges the prevalence of humoral theory in previous scholarship regarding popular notions of sickness and health. The chapter shows that people described themselves as ill and 'incapacitated' as a way of emphasising that their bodies were of less use to them for purposes of work. Corresponding to illness and incapacity were specific measures of abledness, in relation to which a person's varied ability to perform normal routines were assessed. It is thus argued that notions of health were based on people's reliance upon their bodies for purposes of subsistence, and, in conclusion, that people embraced a functional understanding of both ill and good health.

Keywords: early modern household, body, illness, disability, capacity to work

Introduction

At a 1692 court session in Snevringe, a small village outside of the town Västerås, farmer Anders Larsson sued farmhand Olof Nilsson for having breached their employment contract. According to their agreement, Olof was supposed to work for Anders for about four months. However, Olof had only fulfilled his duties for six weeks. In his defense, Olof explained that he had fallen ill and thus had been too weak to perform the tasks expected of him. Anders reproached Olof and stated that he had not demanded Olof to exceed his abilities when working for him. Anders added that Olof, despite his current, frail condition, should at least have been able to thresh grain.

Eyice, M. and C. Forss (eds.), *Health and Society in Early Modern Sweden*.
Taylor & Francis Group 2024
DOI 10.5117/9789463724296_CH02

The court verdict was that Olof should either return his salary in lieu of unfulfilled weeks of work to Anders, or return to work for him for the remaining nine weeks, as stipulated in the original agreement.[1]

The case referred to above offers insights into a typical breach of contract negotiations between a farmer and a farmhand in seventeenth-century Sweden, such as it might unfold in a case of a breach of contract. But it also informs us about how ordinary people in early modern Sweden could use concepts of illness, impairment, and bodily ability in everyday contexts, and more importantly, what meanings were given to these concepts.[2]

The aim of this chapter is twofold: first, to investigate how men and women of early modern Swedish households experienced and interpreted the body as ill, incapacitated, or healthy; second, to discuss what these interpretations reveal about the socioeconomic demands that were related to being able-bodied in this society. Throughout the chapter, I argue that people embraced a functional understanding of both good and ill health, which took as its point of departure a person's need to make a living through the labour of one's body. To some extent, this functional understanding stands in contrast to scientific or medical explanatory frameworks emphasised in historical scholarship.

Previous studies on popular notions and experiences of the early modern body in sickness and health can, when somewhat simplified, be organised into two camps. Several works of medical history from below have, on the one hand, proved that lay people interpreted various diseases as the result of imbalanced or discontinued flows of the four humours. In other words, the persistence of the humoral framework of Galen has been highlighted. The prevalence of this framework was, according to some historians, particularly enduring among the broader strata of early modern European society, not least since it was easy to combine with various magical ways of diagnosing and curing diseases.[3] To most early modern people, this view supposedly continued to be the main frame of reference for experiences of ill health, even after humoral imbalance ceased to be the dominant medical explanation for sickness. Modifying the emphasis placed on the reception of this antique

1 Riksarkivet (RA), Svea Hovrätt, Advokatfiskalens arkiv EXIe:2262, Snevringe häradsrätt, 10 April 1682.

2 In other words, this study is concerned with the same kind of local scene discussed in Miettinen's chapter in this volume.

3 See, e.g., Porter and Porter, *In Sickness and in Health*; Labouvie, 'Der Leib als Medium'; Jütte, *Geschichte der alternativen Medizin*, 68– 78; Wynne Smith, '"An Account of an Unaccountable Distemper,"' 462–463. For discussions of deviations within the humoral framework, see however Duden, *The Woman Beneath the Skin*, 104–179; Rublack, 'Fluxes.'

tradition, other scholarship has drawn attention to how people explained and interpreted illness within the framework of an ontological understanding, which existed alongside the humoral one. According to this stance, illnesses could be understood in terms of disease entities which in various ways had entered the body and made it sick.[4] Generally, when studied as an illness experiencing subject, the early modern body has been characterised either in terms of an 'open' and 'humoral' entity, or as an 'open' but primarily a 'monistic' one, as suggested by Michael Stolberg.[5]

However, similar designations are probably determined by the fact that the experiential aspects of illness, for the most part, have been approached through medical sources – albeit frequently ego-documents, such as patients' diaries or correspondences between patients and doctors. It can be assumed that the accounts of illness that surface in these types of sources have been adapted to the medical contexts they are part of. It is, consequently, quite possible that alternative frameworks for experiencing, interpreting, and describing illness – which were rooted in people's everyday conditions rather than in medical traditions – have been bypassed. For instance, although Stolberg purports to investigate experiences of the ill body from a popular perspective, he does so through a somewhat misrepresentative approach by focusing on sources representing educated nobles and burghers. He defends this approach by claiming that there are no available sources where people from the lower social strata give detailed accounts of their experiences.[6] However, as the case discussed in the opening of the chapter makes evident – and as will become apparent in what follows– this is not quite accurate. In court hearings, ordinary people spoke of illness and health, and at times at length. And they did so in ways not obviously related to a common medical understanding, but instead diverged in important ways from the dominant medical view. By highlighting this practical engagement and understanding of the body, this chapter will thus advance our knowledge of what it meant to be dependent upon one's body in the early modern period.

Scrutinising sources other than medical accounts for a history of illness and health can be productive, and has recently been demonstrated by Olivia Weisser in her work on early modern English petitions for parish relief. By studying the experiential aspects of illness in these sources, Weisser shows that poor people downplayed Galenic notions of illness,

4 Jütte, *Ärzte, Heiler und Patienten*, 124–125; Stolberg, *Experiencing Illness*, 23–33.

5 Stolberg, 'Der gesunde Leib,' 40.

6 Stolberg, *Experiencing Illness*, 13–14.

and instead presented themselves in terms of victims of various accidents. She concludes that this was a strategic way of shifting responsibility from lifestyle choices to, among other things, the hazards of work.[7] For historians seeking to uncover non-medical notions of illness, it is, evidently, worthwhile to approach the subject through sources that are not obviously filtered by medical frameworks. But since petitioners needed to be accepted as deserving of parish support, they needed to present themselves in as pitiable terms as possible. And as Steve Hindle has concluded in his study on the micro-politics of early modern poor relief, petitioners were well versed in notions of Christian duty and paternalistic care.[8] A certain rhetoric of supplication can accordingly be expected to have made the sources bend towards specific moral aspects of illness, at the expense of its more mundane and practical features.

In order to elude this bias, this chapter's discussion primarily relies on court records, more specifically on investigations into magical healing, breaches of contract, and violent crimes. These court documents should prove fruitful since they contain statements that capture themes of relevance, in which notions of sickness and health can be placed centrestage, or simply be alluded to in passing.[9] A further advantage of these sources is their provenance. The lower courts (*ting*) in early modern Sweden were social arenas where everyday conflicts of all sorts were negotiated and resolved. Ordinary men and women not only attended court proceedings as spectators, but to a great extent also actively participated as litigants or as witnesses. They have accordingly left relevant textual traces.[10] Finally, statements in court records can be approached as statements that remain within the scope of an understanding of the world that the informer shares with his or her peers.[11] As such, court records can give insights into notions of sickness and health that were not necessarily filtered by medical understandings nor the rhetoric of supplication, but instead were rooted in peoples' everyday situations. How, then, did men and women describe ill bodies in court?

7 Weisser, *Ill Composed*, 159–180.

8 Hindle, *On the Parish?*, 365.

9 For a discussion of the assumptions serving as guiding principles for the collection of sources, see Runesson, *Blod, kött och tårar*, 37–41. For a discussion on men escaping from naval service, which suggests that cases investigating them are useful sources for this study, see AnnaSara Hammar, *Mellan kaos och kontroll*, 56–58, 178–186.

10 As an institution, the lower courts were social arenas that could fulfil various functions for people, why they made use of them for different purposes. See Österberg and Sogner, eds., *People Meet the Law*.

11 Dulong, *Le témoin oculaire*, 16–18, 56, 185–187.

Illness as incapacity

When people accounted for themselves or others as ill in legal contexts, they commonly characterised illness in terms of various physical deficiencies. These deficiencies were not always specified, but general characteristics were weakness and impotence.[12] For instance, when Agnes Påhlsdotter had to provide reasons for her absence from church one Sunday, a woman who testified in Agnes's defence told how she had noticed, from Agnes's posture, that she had been 'ill and powerless.'[13] A further characteristic of these types of illness accounts is that men and women tended to emphasise that they were ill because they were restricted in their mobility, in that they lacked the ability to move either a specific body part or their bodies as a whole. Thus, when Peder Larsson accused Helfred i Rådhammar of having placed a magic spell on his wife, he described his wife's state in terms of being primarily one of constrained movements. As a consequence of this magical assault, she could 'neither grab with her hands nor walk with her legs.'[14] Similarly, in another case of magic sorcery, Margareta Pehrsdotter described herself as ill due to her inability to move 'any one of her limbs.'[15]

Following from their inabilities to move for different reasons, ill people were often stated to be confined to bed, and as such they needed care from their families or other members of their households.[16] Being bedridden could also be put forth as a reason for people failing to appear in court. This was the case for Kerstin Andersdotter, who was supposed to testify against another woman in an investigation into claims of magic. Kerstin's husband, along with a couple of her neighbours, testified that she was indeed confined to bed and thus unable to bring herself to the court hearing.[17] If immobility was an important characteristic of illness, the ability to move

12 See, e.g., Ericsson, ed., *Vadstena stads äldsta tänkeböcker 1577–1610*, 349–374; Landsarkivet i Uppsala (ULA), Kopparbergs och Säters län (utom Säters socken) och Österdalarne tingslags häradsrättsarkiv A AI:4, Leksands, Åls och Bjursås häradsrätt, 8 December 1714.

13 Richardsson, ed., *Revsunds tingslags domboksprotokoll 1649–1700*, 160.

14 ULA, Askers häradsrättsarkiv AI:I, Laga ting i Asker, 3 June, 1633. See also ULA, Våla häradsrättsarkiv AIA:14, Våla häradsrätt, 15 February 1754.

15 ULA, Österdalarne och Gagnefs sockens tingslags häradsrättsarkiv AI:2, Rättviks häradsrätt, 9 December 1663. See also RA, Svea Hovrätt, Advokatfiskalens arkiv EXIe:1778, Örebro häradsrätt, 17 July 1632.

16 ULA, Kopparbergs och Säters län (utom Säters socken) och Österdalarne tingslags häradsrättsarkiv AI:16, Stora Tuna häradsrätt, 25 May 1722. See also Jütte, *Ärzte, Heiler und Patienten*, 163–164.

17 ULA, Kopparbergs och Säters län (utom Säters socken) och Österdalarne tingslags häradsrättsarkiv A AI:16, Stora Tuna häradsrätt, 25 October 1722.

one's body parts again, perhaps even to the extent of being able to get out of bed, was perceived as a common sign of being on the road to recovery. Margareta Pehrsdotter, for example, accounted for her progressive process of recovery as the gradual onset of mobility of her limbs.[18] And as Jon Strett gave testimony regarding his dying sister's final days, he related her brief and transient recovery with reference to her having been confined to bed all Sunday, but that she had then been able to walk from Monday to Friday, when she, finally, laid down again.[19]

That ill people were confined to bed should perhaps not come as a surprise, but neither should it be taken as an empty truism. Taking to bed carried specific meanings in early modern Europe. Already in their classic study of patients in early modern England, Dorothy and Roy Porter showed that writing of themselves as bedridden was a way for people to highlight the social consequences of illness and of demarcating that they, as sick people, were excluded from the community of the healthy. Essentially, taking to one's bed was a way of communicating that one accepted the role of being a sick person. In turn, this brought about a temporary hiatus from everyday responsibilities, which could reverse certain social hierarchies, and as such be empowering for the ill person.[20] Accordingly, for poor people petitioning for relief, stressing confinement to bed could, of course, be an efficient strategy of presenting themselves as worthy of pity and deserving of help.[21] Be that as it may, in the context of the the empirical evidence discussed here, I would rather suggest that statements of being bedridden should be interpreted as people either conveying that they were severely ill (as was the case for the dying sister mentioned above), or as a way, more generally, of highlighting the ramifications of being ill and its impact on one's ability to work.

It is probably in this second sense that we should understand the fact that in Swedish court records, women who were expected to soon give birth as well as those who had recently given birth, all could be referred to as ill. Both states of being did, after all, require that women took to bed, and following from this, they could not perform the tasks expected of them as wives or handmaids. To give but one example from a court investigation, when Marit Persdotter was accused of infanticide – in spite of the fact

18 ULA, Österdalarne och Gagnefs sockens tingslags häradsrättsarkiv AI:2, Rättviks häradsrätt, 9 December 1663.

19 *Vadstena stads äldsta tänkeböcker 1577–1610*, 291. See also ULA, Uppsala kämnärsrätts arkiv AI:24, 3 July 1752.

20 Porter and Porter, *In Sickness and in Health*, 192–200.

21 Weisser, *Ill Composed*, 173.

that she was married – her husband testified that she had in fact suffered a proper, if yet curious, stillbirth. He could assert that she had been 'sick in childbed.'[22] The fact that being pregnant or recently having given birth could be described in terms of illness illustrates the breadth of the concept of illness. Illness was clearly an umbrella term for various states of being, in which peoples' bodies differed from their normal or usual ways of being and moving.[23]

Related to this broad inclusiveness of modes of sickness is the fact that when people described or invoked states of being ill, they rarely named specific diseases.[24] It was instead the experiences and, as already mentioned, the different consequences of being ill that were placed centre stage. Again, the investigation into the sudden onset of Margareta Pehrsdotter's illness is particularly informative as the way she characterised her illness is both illustrative and explanatory. Along with several others, Margareta accused a woman called Håll Karin of having made her ill some years earlier. As Margareta explained how she realised that she had fallen ill, she recounted that she had sensed how a disease entity had subjugated her body and its abilities. She also related the detrimental effects of this. To her, it had been 'as if someone had held her in a grip so that she could not move and only barely cry for help.'[25] This tendency to focus on specific experiential or consequential aspects of illness could, of course, simply indicate that many diseases lacked established designations or that it was, for various reasons, superfluous to specifically name illnesses in the context of the court proceedings. It could additionally, as Weisser concludes with regards to similar observations in petitions of the poor, be due to the fact that what mattered for the afflicted was to be accepted as persons in need of support.[26] However, since the rationale behind petitioning for support and testifying in

22 Hellbom, ed., *Tingsprotokoll för Njurunda* 2, 303. The 'curious' aspect of the case is that Marit was described as having given birth, yet no child had been born, as she and her husband claimed that what emanated from her body was merely a small cloth of blood. For a further testimony in which pregnancy is described in terms of illness, see Edling, ed., *Östra härads i Njudung dombok 1602–1605*, 48.

23 Compare umbrella terms for madness and insanity discussed in Miettinen's chapter in this volume.

24 There were of course deviations from this norm. Fever and epileptic diseases were regularly named, probably because they repercussed also on the mind and thus often gave rise to erratic behavior. See Runesson, *Blod, kött och tårar*, 86–87.

25 ULA, Österdalarne och Gagnefs sockens tingslags häradsrättsarkiv AI:2, Rättviks häradsrätt, 9 December 1663. For a similar description, also in an investigation into magic, see RA, Svea Hovrätt, Advokatfiskalens arkiv E XI e:1130, Rönö häradsrätt, 11 December 1706.

26 Weisser, *Ill Composed*, 172.

court were somewhat different, yet another way of interpreting this becomes possible. I argue that the lack of designations for diseases is related to the fact that the experienes and consequences of illness, in the sense of being incapable of functioning normally, was crucial to the understanding of illness studied here. Moreover, I argue that this way of interpreting bodily change was embedded in early modern societal demands of being able-bodied so as to be capable to support oneself.

Incapacity as disability to work

The inclination of early modern men and women to communicate the experiential effects of being ill sheds light on why the line between the concepts of disease and injury were blurred. In fact, people used the concept of illness to include states of being that we today understand in terms of injuries and various inabilities. The interrogation into the death of farmer Anders Eriksson illustrates this. His wife Anna Israelsdotter testified that after Anders had been severely beaten by bailiff Mattias Trost, he 'contracted a disease that resulted in death.'[27] A vicar had visited Anders on his deathbed, and testified in court to Anders's final words. Shortly before he passed away, Anders stated that the bailiff's violent assault was the reason for him having 'become ill and incapacitated.' Along the same lines, as another interrogation into manslaughter makes clear, a kick in the groin could be termed a disease, and the stricken person described as ill.[28] Injured or wounded individuals could be described as ill, since they too were unable to function and move as they normally did or were expected to. Consequently, the terms for illness and injury could be used interchangeably in this type of context, or be singularly expressed by the key word 'incapacitated' (Swe. *Ofärdig*) as cited in the passage above.

The concept *ofärdig* is a negation of *färdig*, that is, of being able to fare or move. According to the historical dictionary, *ofärdig* could either refer to a person (or an animal) lacking one or several of his or her bodily abilities, or to an object that was out of order and hence of less or of no use.[29] When used in early modern Swedish courts, these two meanings of the concept

27 Wikström, ed., *Stockholms stads tänkeböcker från år 1592, vol. 10. 1618*, quotations at 377 and 380.

28 Landsarkivet i Vadstena (VLA), Göta hovrätt EVAA:44, Göta hovrätts protokoll, 3 November 1654. See also RA, Svea Hovrätt, Advokatfiskalens arkiv E XI e:4, Närdingshundra häradsrätt, 5 October 1683.

29 Cf. *Svenska Akademiens Ordbok*: *Ofärdig*.

seem to have been merged. 'Incapacity' was commonly inferred when people described specific body parts that were no longer functional in their normal manner, and which were therefore, importantly, of less or of no use to the afflicted person. In particular, interrogations held regarding magic assaults that resulted in bodily harm exemplify the merged meanings of this word.

For instance, in the village of Asker in 1645, an older woman named Elin (no surname is stated in the court record) was accused of having performed magic and made several people in the village fall ill. The farmer Olof Bengtsson was one of the litigants who accused Elin. He claimed that she had cast a spell on his horse, which had made the horse unruly and resulted in him falling from it. From falling to the ground, his arm was broken and became 'incapacitated.' Since the investigative hearings against Elin were lengthy, Olof was asked to repeat his case in court. But the second time he was heard, Olof described his incapacitated condition and its onset in another way. Now he maintained that Elin hade made him suffer from a deteriorating sickness, which had gradually spread inside him and subjugated more and more parts of his body ('alt mehr och mehr, hafuer sigh förökat').[30] For Olof, falling from a horse and damaging his arm was clearly more or less the same as becoming ill from some disease entity. The truth of the matter was, probably, that his arm was no longer functional, and that he was suffering. Similarly, in 1687 Anders Eriksson accused Sofia Welamsdotter of having cast a spell on his son. Anders presented his son as 'incapacitated,' since the young boy could no longer move his lower limbs. Interestingly, he placed his son's present condition in contrast to his ordinary state of being, as Anders maintained that the boy was usually 'healthy and capable of walking and running.'[31] I will return to this way of assessing illness according to individual standards of bodily movement, but what is particularly worth emphasising in accounts of incapacity as these is the notion that a healthy body should consist of functioning body parts in order to be functioning as a whole. When used to describe states of being ill or inhibited, the concept of incapacity thus comes close to both historical and contemporary definitions of disability, as these descriptions were and are also often formulated in terms of negations.[32] In the sources studied here, these negations signalled that body parts were not accessible and functioning as previously. Beyond such concrete references,

30 ULA, Askers häradsrätt AIa:1, Laga ting i Asker, 30 April 1645.

31 ULA, Vendels häradsrättsarkiv A AI:2, Vendels häradsrätt, 15 October 1687. For further evidence, see statements in passing in Hjelmberg ed., *Stora Malms sockenstämmoprotokoll II 1728–1741*, 114.

32 In his historical overview, Henri-Jacques Stiker points to the use of terms such as 'malformation,' 'infirm,' 'incapacité.' See Stiker, *Corps infirmes et sociétés*, 48, 118, 220.

however, these specific uses of words call attention to how important it was for people to have able bodies for purposes of everyday subsistence.

In early modern Sweden, all people, except children, were legally required to work. If one could not work, one was eligible for relief and subsistence aid but this required proof of one's inability to work.[33] Recent studies on work and working relations within households have highlighted that the men and women making up this economic unit were devoting most of the day and of the year working together. The maintenance and survival of a household depended on the ability of each member to constantly perform different tasks. Being able to work was thus a precondition for people trying to make a living for themselves and for those they supported.[34] But being able to perform work did also carry other meanings. By taking part in the subsistence of the household, men and women proved themselves to be useful, and could accordingly be recognised as honourable members of society.[35] Illness in terms of inability to work can accordingly be understood as departing from people needing their bodies to function as a means to provide for themselves, but also in order to be included in the community. This being the case, I suggest that the wide-ranging concept of illness – along with the blurred lines between illness and injury –was rooted in the different tasks people needed to perform with their bodies.

Thus far, I have discussed cases in which it was not specified how illness in terms of incapacity inhibited afflicted men and women from working. It was, however, probably implied in many cases. Consequently, it should come as no surprise that a person with a 'spoiled health'– as witnesses described Kerstin Perdotter's state of being after Olof Ersson Swan had put a spell on her – was not able to work as she was used to.[36] Yet more intriguing is the fact that afflicted persons often named the relation between specific body parts that were incapacitated as a result of illness and injury, and themselves as incapacitated persons with subsequent inabilities to perform expected tasks and responsibilities.

33 See discussion in Ling, *Konsten att försörja sig*, 11–35.

34 Lindström, Fiebranz, and Rydén, 'The Diversity of Work,' 33–35, 49. For a discussion of the ubiquity of work in a European perspective, see Whittle, 'A Critique of Approaches to "Domestic Work."' See also Widmalm's chapter in this volume.

35 Hassan Jansson, Fiebranz, and Östman, 'Constitutive Tasks: Performances of Hierarchy and Identity,' 151–153. Compare Gray, 'Petitioning for Survival.' On the performativity of performing work for others, see also Uppenberg, *I husbondens bröd och arbete*, 256.

36 ULA, Kopparbergs och Säters län (utom Säters socken) och Österdalarne tingslags häradsrättsarkiv AI:15, Rättviks häradsrätt, 20 March 1721. For a case of a man prevented from making fences due to illness, see RA, Justitierevisionens arkiv, Utslagshandlingar i besvärs– och ansökningsmål 17 juni 1776 (no. 50–80), no. 56 1/2 Utslagshandling, 17 June 1776.

For instance, when the maid Anna Larsdotter – along with the aforementioned Kerstin Persdotter – accused Olof Ersson Swan for having made her ill by way of a magic spell, she emphasised that his spell had resulted in her becoming restricted in moving her fingers as she was normally able to. This, in turn, impaired her ability to work, which two members of her household testified was the case. In confirming Anna's statement, they put her current state of being in contrast to her usual way of being 'industrious in her work.'[37] In a similar way, when Märit Olsdotter accused Peder Ersson Bång of having raped her, his violence towards her was presented as evidence against him, not least since it had left parts of her body not functioning as before. According to Märit, Peder had injured her right arm and hand to the extent that they were incapacitated, and of less use to her in her work. The farmer Nils Jacobsson, for whom Märit worked, asserted this. He corroborated that shortly after the assault, as Märit was supposed to help him carry hay, he had to reproach her for working too slowly, whereupon she had explained that it was because she had been assaulted by Bång.[38] Finally, when wife Gertrud Jonsdotter accused mercenary Erik Ersson Wästman of domestic violence, she testified that he twice had beaten her severely on her right arm and shoulder, leaving her 'incapacitated [...] to do any work.'[39] We can assume that both victims in these last two cases were right-handed, as both testimonies speak to the importance of being able to use one's dominant hand and arm. But more importantly, the testimonies of Märit and Gertrud support the conclusion that the blurring of lines between illness and injury were determined by the fact that, either way, the afflicted persons were disabled in their (normal) corporeality, so that they could not normally employ their bodily capacities in their work.

Although inability to work was important to convey for incapacitated people, being incapacitated needed not be a complete bodily redefinition of a person's state of being. Notions of certain quantifying assessments of abledness were in circulation, which in turn illustrate the elasticity of early modern incapacity. These quantifying assessments were made relevant in cases of disputed inabilities to work. For example, when Per Olofsson informed the court of his brother's state of being slightly ill, he specified that even though he had not been particularly healthy of late, he had never been bedridden. At least for the most part, he had managed to 'perform his

37 ULA, Kopparbergs och Säters län (utom Säters socken) och Österdalarne tingslags häradsarkiv AI:15, Rättviks häradsrätt, 20 March 1721.

38 Tegen, ed., *Hallens tingslags domboksprotokoll 1648–1700*, 138–139, 148–149.

39 Tegen, ed., *Hallens tingslags domboksprotokoll 1648–1700*, 122.

tasks.[40] In another case, the former crofter Pär Pärsson explained that his capacity for work had become diminished after he had become sick from a hernia, yet he specified that this condition only made him unable to work most days, as he could still perform some tasks on 'his healthy days.'[41] Yet another assessment of abledness was particularly recurring in cases in which men serving in the navy, who were temporarily dismissed for purposes of recovery, were accused for having travelled too far away from their crew. For instance, after the boatswain Mats Jansson Dahl became sick, he had been allowed leave of absence for a short period of time, yet he was reproached for having gone all the way home to his village.[42] Returning home seems to have been reserved for the severely ill, but not for subordinates who were expected to soon be able to serve again.

Crucial to the breadth and inclusiveness of the concept of incapacity – along with those of illness and injury – was the way that people could be evaluated according to corresponding assessments of capability, in relation to which their capacity for carrying out alternative tasks could be weighed. These nuances become evident when attention is paid to what work people were able to do, despite of their illnesses or injuries, that is, when work tasks were adapted to the varied functioning abilities of their bodies. A case of a poor labourer who reported being robbed implies this type of occurrence. In 1690, a former farmhand named Nils (no family name was registered in the court records) appeared before the court in the town of Örebro, after he had been robbed of his few possessions. In passing, he mentioned that he was incapacitated (albeit in an unspecified way), which is why he, for some time, had been making his living from selling bread and fruit in a tiny shed, rather than performing farmhand work, as he did previously .[43] Similarly, a resident registration document (Swe. *mantalslängd*) from Stockholm in 1740 specifies that Hans Hindrichsson Skog, who was also incapacitated in an undisclosed way, now made his living from teaching children how to read.[44] And after Peder Eriksson Blom had only partly recovered from a period of illness and confinement to his sickbed, he maintained that he

40 RA, Justitierevisionens arkiv, utslagshandlingar i besvärs– och ansökningsmål 56 1/2 Utslagshandling, 17 June 1776.

41 Hjelmberg, ed., *Stora Malms sockenstämmoprotokoll II 1728–1741*, 112. See also Hansson, ed., *Hammerdals tingslags domboksprotokoll 1649–1690*, 126.

42 Krigsarkivet (KA), Flottans arkiv, Amiralitetsrättens arkiv 1673–1716 A:2, 6 July 1685.

43 ULA, Örebro rådhusrätt och magistrats arkiv A1A:15, Örebro rådhusrätt, 26 February 1690.

44 Stockholms stadsarkiv (SSA), Överståthållarämbetet för uppbördsärenden G1BA:17:4, Stockholms mantalslängder, Qvart:t Träskbacken. For a discussion of blind people making their living from teaching in early modern Sweden, see Bondestam, *Människans metamorfos*, 210.

was unfit to take up a position as a boatswain again (as he was supposed to do), and instead wanted to continue supporting himself by selling beer and animal fat at a market in Stockholm, together with his wife.[45] This tendency of adjusting one's strategy of subsistence according to one's bodily abilities is in fact particularly evident in cases of legal investigations into escaped naval seamen, who had abandoned their duties for reasons of ill health. When Per Eriksson Nässla fell ill, he had escaped from his employment as naval spinner and fled to a village in northern Sweden, where he had assumed a position as a boatswain. When tracked down and accused of abandoning his duties, he defended himself by explaining that, as a consequence of his illness, he was not able to perform spinning work, yet could well manage the tasks expected of a boatswain.[46]

Following a redefinition of bodily functioning, an ill person who was accustomed to one type of work could, evidently, adjust his or her means of support by performing another type of work. Varying degrees of illness and incapacity thus seem to have been assessed and acknowledged according to the sick person's varying (in)ability to work. On the one hand, this resonates with previous research on popular notions of sickness and health, where emphasis has been placed on the elasticity of these concepts. Medical history from the perspective of patients has shown that as patients, people had their individual humoral dispositions that served as reference points when assessing their health. The medical term for this was 'complexion.'[47] But on the other hand, the empirical evidence points in another direction. Rather than making references to complexions when conceptualising bodily change, men and women as litigants, defendants, and witnesses rather made references to how their specific capabilities to work had changed. As such, the uncovered notions of illness and health were relative and individual, but in ways differing from the notion of complexion as an expression of one's disposition, as people could also depart from their specific capabilities for work when they made sense of bodily change due to illness.

These findings run counter to the conclusions drawn by Irina Metzler in her study of disability and work in Medieval Europe, as she states that illness and disability were 'two distinct conceptual and cultural categories.'[48] Early modern Swedish court cases, however, suggest that illness and disability

45 KA, Flottans arkiv, Amiralitetsrättens arkiv 1673–1716 A:2, 21 January 1685.

46 KA, Flottans arkiv, Amiralitetsrättens protokoll A:1, 5/4 1673. For a case in which four men stood accused of this, see Amiralitetsrättens protokoll A:1, 7 May 1673.

47 See, e.g., Lindemann, *Medicine and Society*, 84–120; compare Jütte, *Ärzte, Heiler, und Patienten*, 53–55.

48 Metzler, *A Social History of Disability*, 199–205, quotation at 204.

overlapped. The results of this chapter are thus more in line with those of historian of military medicine Geoffrey L. Hudson. In his study on how British veterans sought support after they had been disabled from serving in battle, Hudson has similarly found that ex-servicemen stressed that their disabilities prevented them from being able to work. Hudson thus concludes that scholars who argue that the category 'disability' was a medical construct are on the wrong track. His empirical evidence from military medical practice and veterans' petitions for pensions suggests instead that early modern 'disability' was a social and political construct, which emanated from veterans' struggle for support and recognition.[49] Departing from the court cases discussed throughout this chapter, I would – with some caution, however – concur with Hudson's statement that 'the only recognised "disability" was the disability to work.'[50] It remains for future studies to investigate the discourse of incapacity in other contexts, such as in relation to sexual impotence.

Consistent with the line of argument pursued in this chapter, descriptions of recovery from illness in the studied sources not only implied to regain health, but also, ultimately, to become fit for work again. The account of blacksmith Mårten Martinell supports this point. After he had suffered a stroke (Swe. *Slag*), he was cured by a healer living outside of Uppsala. In court, a maid who knew Mårten testified, and in so doing, she corroborated that, after having received treatment, Mårten had gradually become better and had finally been able to return to work ('han blev därefter mer och mer bättre, att han ock nu kan arbeta').[51] Similarly, after farmhand Hans Persson had recuperated from an undisclosed illness, he could return to work as an iron-maker for Måns Christersson, and serve his full term of employment.[52]

In essence, recovery was often described as a return to a former and normal state of being, that is, to the time before incapacity had redefined a person's existence and when one's body functioned and could be used

49 Hudson, 'Arguing Disability,' 109–110, 133, 116–117.

50 Hudson, 'Arguing Disability,' 116.

51 ULA, Lövsta häradsrättsarkiv AI:1, Laga ting i Lövsta, 16 September 1714. Similarly, Erik Abrahamsson Abrill was described as 'healthy and capable'; see Larsen and Rauø, eds., *Dombok Torneå Lappmark. Jukkasjärvi og Enontekis tinglag 1727–1732*, 95. See also ULA, Kopparbergs och Näsgårds län samt Säters och Tuna tingslags häradsrättsarkiv AI:13, Hedemora häradsrätt, 11 October 1669.

52 ULA, Snevringe häradsrättsarkiv AIA:4, Snevringe häradsrätt, 2 October 1680. For a similar case, see ULA, Kopparbergs och Näsgårds län samt Säters och Tuna tingslags häradsrättsarkiv AI:13, Folkare häradsrätt, 15 October 1669.

purposefully for everyday activities.[53] Illness as incapacity corresponded with notions of recovery from illness in terms of regained abilities to work again. All in all, these conclusions align with both historical and contemporary studies of disability, according to which notions of inability and negations of abledness shed light on how bodies are and were valued with regards to their abilities.[54] In short, 'incapacity' was a useful hypernym to describe people with ill and injured bodies and body parts, as it was effective in communicating that they were thereby of less use within the household economy.

Conclusions

This chapter has examined how men and women in early modern Sweden described themselves and others as ill, impaired, or healthy in legal contexts. The chapter's aim has been to understand what meanings were embedded in non-medical and everyday notions of these concepts, so as to further our knowledge of the significance of having a well-functioning body in this society.

The chapter began by calling attention to the breadth and inclusiveness of the concept of illness that was in circulation in early modern Swedish society. It is evident that people understood themselves and others as ill when, for different reasons, their bodies were weakened and did not function as they normally did. In comparison with what previous scholarship on popular notions of sickness and health has found, allusions to humoral theory are rare in the sources examined in this chapter. When presenting information in court, people did not comply with the dominant medical discourse of the times. Instead, they kept within the scope of everyday notions of physiology that they shared with one another. A key word that was often invoked when referring to bodies or body parts that were ill and out of function was 'incapacitated.' Ill men and women were described as incapacitated when they could not utilise their physical capacities as usually was the case, and hence could not support themselves by working as they normally did. Parallel to the notion of 'incapacity'

53 For a variety of examples of this, see Runesson, *Blod, kött och tårar*, 96–97. Weisser, too, has found evidence of this way of assessing the severity of illness and progression of recovery in relation to people's abilities to work, however from the perspectives of ministers, merchants, book sellers, and tax collectors. Compare Weisser, *Ill Composed*, 113–114.

54 For theoretical points of departure, see Campbell, *Contours of Ableism*, 3–15. For sociohistorical perspectives, compare Turner, 'Approaching Anomalous Bodies.'

was the acceptance of certain quantitative assessments of abledness to determine variations of bodily capabilities. Thus, persons with redefined bodily dispositions could adapt to their new circumstances and make their living from performing other types of work. Along similar lines, the chapter furthermore indicates that people understood recovery from illness in terms of returning to former states of being, that is, to the time before illnesses redefined their bodies and they could be used purposefully for work again.

This particular understanding of illness and health, to which ordinary people adhered when they made sense of their ailing bodies outside of the era's medical discourse, is more in line with current research on early modern forms of disability than with traditional medical history. Rather than attesting to the persistence of humoral theory, the notions of ill and good health examined here suggest that, as members of households, ordinary people embraced a functional and pragmatic way of interpreting the body. This understanding was rooted in the social conditions of the times, and determined people's dependence upon their bodies. They needed healthy bodies to be able to work.

Bibliography

Archival sources

Riksarkivet Marieberg, Stockholm (RA)
Justitierevisionens arkiv, utslagshandlingar i besvärs– och ansökningsmål.

Svea Hovrätts arkiv
Advokatfiskalens arkiv
EXIe:1778, Örebro häradsrätt 17/7 1632.
E XI e:1130, Rönö häradsrätt 11/12 1706.
E XI e:4, Närdingshundra häradsrätt 5/10 1683.

Krigsarkivet Arninge, Stockholm (KA)
Flottans arkiv
Amiralitetsrättens arkiv 1673–1716 A:1–2.

Stockholms stadsarkiv (SSA)
Överståthållarämbetet för uppbördsärenden G1BA:17:4, Stockholms mantal-längder, Qvart:t Träskbacken.

Landsarkivet i Vadstena (VLA)
Göta hovrätts arkiv EVAA:44.

Landsarkivet i Uppsala (ULA)
Askers häradsrättsarkiv AI:I.
Kopparbergs och Näsgårds län samt Säters och Tuna tingslags häradsrättsarkiv.
AI:13, Folkare häradsrättsarkiv.
AI:13, Hedemora häradsrättsarkiv.
Kopparbergs och Säters län (utom Säters socken) och Österdalarne tingslags häradsrättsarkiv.
A AI:4, Leksands, Åls och Bjursås häradsrättsarkiv.
AI:15, Rättviks häradsrättsarkiv.
AI:16, Stora Tuna häradsrättsarkiv.
Lövsta häradsrättsarkiv AI:1.
Snevringe häradsrättsarkiv AIA:4.
Vendels häradsrättsarkiv A AI:2.
Våla häradsrättsarkiv AIA:14.
Örebro rådhusrätt och magistrats arkiv A1A:15.
Österdalarne och Gagnefs sockens tingslags häradsrättsarkiv AI:2, Rättviks häradsrättsarkiv.

Printed works

Edling, Nils, ed. *Östra härads i Njudung dombok 1602–1605*. Stockholm: Almqvist & Wiksell, 1965.

Ericsson, Georg J. V., ed. *Vadstena stads äldsta tänkeböcker 1577–1610*. Uppsala: Almqvist & Wiksell, 1952.

Hansson, George, ed. *Hammerdals tingslags domboksprotokoll 1649–1690*. Östersund: Landsarkivet i Östersund & Jämtlands läns fornskriftsällskap, 2011.

Hellbom, Algot, ed. *Tingsprotokoll för Njurunda 2: Ur Medelpads domböcker 1673–1699*. Sundsvall: Medelpads fornminnesförening, 1983.

Hjelmberg, Hilding, ed. *Stora Malms sockenstämmoprotokoll II 1728–1741*. Katrineholm: Katrineholms hembygdsförening, 1959.

Larsen, Dag A., and Rauø, Kåre. *Dombok Torneå Lappmark: Jukkasjärvi og Enontekis tinglag 1727–1732*. Finnsnes: Lenvik bygdemuseum, 1994.

Richardsson, Ingegerd, ed. *Revsunds tingslags domboksprotokoll 1649–1700*. Östersund: Landsarkivet i Östersund & Jämtlands läns fornskriftsällskap, 2011.

Tegen, Andreas, ed. *Hallens tingslags domboksprotokoll 1648–1700*. Östersund: Landsarkivet i Östersund & Jämtlands läns fornskriftsällskap, 2020.

Wikström, Lars, ed. *Stockholms stads tänkeböcker från år 1592*, vol. 10. *1618*. Stockholm: Stockholms stadsarkiv, 1973.

Literature

Bondestam Maja. *Människans metamorfos: Ålder och den mognande kroppens politik, 1580–1850*. Nora: Nya Doxa, 2020.

Campbell, Fiona Kumari. *Contours of Ableism: The Production of Disability and Abledness*. Basingstoke: Palgrave Macmillan, 2009.

Duden, Barbara. *The Woman Beneath the Skin: A Doctor's Patients in Eighteenth-Century Germany*. Translated by Thomas Dunlap. Cambridge, MA: Harvard University Press, 1991.

Dulong, Renaud. *Le témoin oculaire: Les conditions sociales de l'attestation personnelle*. Paris: Éditions de l'École des hautes études en sciences sociales, 1998.

Gray, Louise. 'Petitioning for Survival: Medical Care and Welfare Provision in Early Modern German Hospitals.' *Medicina & storia: Rivista de storia della medicina e della santia* 6 (2003): 26–43.

Hammar, AnnaSara. *Mellan kaos och kontroll: Social ordning i svenska flottan 1670–1716*. Lund: Nordic Academic Press, 2014.

Hassan Jansson, Karin, Rosemarie Fiebranz, and Ann-Catrin Östman. 'Constitutive Tasks: Performances of Hierarchy and Identity.' In *Making a Living, Making a Difference: Gender and Work in Early Modern European Society*, edited by Maria Ågren, 127–158. Oxford: Oxford University Press, 2017.

Hindle, Steve. *On the Parish? The Micro-Politics of Poor Relief in Rural England c. 1550–1750*. Oxford: Clarendon, 2004.

Hudson, Geoffrey L. 'Arguing Disability: Ex-Servicemen's Own Stories in Early Modern England, 1590–1790.' In *Medicine, Madness and Social History: Essays in Honour of Roy Porter*, edited by Roberta Bivins and John V. Pickstone, 104–117. Basingstoke: Palgrave Macmillan, 2007.

Jütte, Robert. *Ärzte, Heiler und Patienten: Medizinischer Alltag in der Frühen Neuzeit*. Munich: Artemis und Winkler, 1991.

Jütte, Robert. *Geschichte der alternativen Medizin. Von der Volksmedizin zu den unkonventionellen Therapien von heute*. Munich: Beck, 1996.

Labouvie, Eva. 'Der Leib als Medium, Raum, Zeichen und Zustand. Zur kulturellen Erfahrung und Selbstwahrnehmung des schwangeren Körpers.' In *Erfahrung als Kategorie der Frühneuzeitgeschichte. Historische Zeitschrift: Beiheft 31*, edited by Paul Münch, 115–126. Munich: Oldenbourg Wissenschaftsverlag, 2001.

Lindemann, Mary. *Medicine and Society in Early Modern Europe*. Cambridge: Cambridge University Press, 2010.

Lindström, Jonas, Rosemarie Fiebranz, and Göran Rydén. 'The Diversity of Work.' In *Making a Living, Making a Difference: Gender and Work in Early Modern European Society*, edited by Maria Ågren, 24–56. Oxford: Oxford University Press, 2017.

Ling, Sofia. *Konsten att försörja sig: Kvinnors arbete i Stockholm 1650–1750*. Stockholm: Stockholmia, 2016.

Metzler, Irina. *A Social History of Disability in the Middle Ages: Cultural Considerations of Physical Impairment*. New York: Routledge, 2013.

Österberg, Eva, and Sølvi Sogner, eds. *People Meet the Law: Control and Conflict-Handling in the Courts. The Nordic Countries in the Post-Reformation and Pre-industrial Period*. Oslo: Universitetsforlaget, 2000.

Porter, Dorothy, and Porter, Roy. *In Sickness and in Health: The British Experience 1650–1850*. London: Fourth Estate, 1988.

Rublack, Ulinka. 'Fluxes: The Early Modern Body and the Emotions.' *History Workshop Journal* 53 (2002): 1–16.

Runesson, Anton. *Blod, kött och tårar: Kroppslig erfarenhet i Sverige ca 1600–1750*. Stockholm: Stockholms universitet, 2021.

Stiker, Henri-Jacques. *Corps infirmes et sociétés: Essais d'anthropologie historique*. Paris: Dunod, 2005.

Stolberg, Michael. *Experiencing Illness and the Sick Body in Early Modern Europe*. Translated by Leonhard Unglaub and Logan Kennedy. Basingstoke: Palgrave Macmillan, 2011.

Stolberg, Michael. 'Der gesunde Leib: Zur Geschichtlichkeit frühneuzeitlicher Körpererfahrung.' In *Erfahrung als Kategorie der Frühneuzeitgeschichte. Historische Zeitschrift: Beiheft 31*, edited by Paul Münch, 37–58. Munich: Oldenbourg Wissenschaftsverlag, 2001.

Svenska Akademiens Ordbok. https://www.saob.se/.

Turner, David M. 'Introduction: Approaching Anomalous Bodies.' In *Social Histories of Disability and Deformity*, edited by David M. Turner and Kevin Stagg, 1–16. London: Routledge, 2006.

Uppenberg, Carolina. *I husbondens bröd och arbete: Kön, makt och kontrakt i det svenska tjänstefolkssystemet 1730–1860*. Gothenburg: Göteborgs universitet, 2018.

Weisser, Olivia. *Ill Composed: Sickness, Gender, and Belief in Early Modern England*. New Haven, CT: Yale University Press, 2015.

Whittle, Jane. 'A Critique of Approaches to "Domestic Work": Women, Work and the Pre-industrial Economy.' *Past & Present* 243, no. 1 (2019): 35–70.

Wynne Smith, Lisa. '"An Account of an Unaccountable Distemper": The Experience of Pain in Early Eighteenth-Century England and France.' *Eighteenth-Century Studies* 41, no. 4 (2008): 459–480.

About the Author

Anton Runesson is a Postdoctoral Researcher at Stockholm University and the University of Strathclyde, Glasgow, working on a project on human-animal relations in early modern Swedish households. His doctoral thesis investigated popular notions of physiology in seventeenth- and eighteenth-century Sweden.

3. The Body in the Bathhouse: Health and Bathing in Early Modern Sweden

Charlotta Forss

Abstract

This study examines what was considered healthy and unhealthy in relation to the early modern Swedish sweat bath culture. Health in the bathhouse, or sauna, was far from straight forward. Instead, an array of factors was understood to work together to determine if a particular bath was healthy for a particular body, at a particular time. By mapping out these complexities, the study brings attention to how different interpretative frameworks and practical circumstance interlinked in the day-to-day determination of what was healthy in the early modern period. While health was a signifier of the good life, it was also understood as situation-dependent, tied to body types and to places.

Keywords: balneology, sauna, bathhouse, history of the body, health, social practice

Introduction

Walking through the streets of early modern Stockholm, a visitor would, sooner rather than later, encounter the sign of a public bathhouse.[1] A set of metal dishes or a bunch of birch tree twigs hung outside a building was a sign that one could take a sweat bath, or sauna, within.[2] Some sweat baths

1 This study is part of my research project on health and morality in the early modern Swedish sweat bath, funded by the Swedish Research Council (2018-06765). I would like to express my particular gratitude to Mari Eyice, Lisa Hellman, Martina Hjertman, Margaret Hunt, Jezzica Israelsson, Joachim Östlund, Lyndal Roper, Karin Sennefelt, and Astrid Wendel-Hansen, who have read and provided valuable feedback on drafts of this study.

2 The specific signs used varied over time and depending on the qualifications of the proprietor. See Hjelt, *Svenska och finska medicinalverkets historia*, 1:222–225.

Eyice, M. and C. Forss (eds.), *Health and Society in Early Modern Sweden*. Taylor & Francis Group 2024
DOI 10.5117/9789463724296_CH03

were large establishments, run by the masters of the city's Bathing Guild.[3] Others were more transitory, illicitly set up and catering to community needs for bathing and socialising. In early modern Sweden (including Finland), there were sweat baths in the cities, in smaller towns and in the countryside. These were places where people met to talk and have a good time. Indeed, nineteenth- and twentieth-century historians and folklorists viewed the sweat bath as an integral part of Nordic medieval and early modern culture.[4] In recent years, however, the bathhouse culture of early modern Sweden has largely been overlooked by historians.[5] This chapter makes a case for reinstating the bathhouse as an integral part of early modern Swedish culture. In particular, in early modern Sweden, a visit to the bathhouse was understood to affect a person's health.

The introduction to this volume contends that 'health' as a concept in early modern Sweden referred both to bodily and mental well-being, and to a broader understanding of a person's prosperity in life. Health was also used as a metaphor in religious, moral, and political conceptions of society.[6] The present chapter complements this broad picture with a focused analysis of what was considered healthy, and unhealthy, in relation to a specific setting: the body in the bathhouse. As we will see, health in the bathhouse was far from obvious. Instead, an array of factors was understood to work together to determine if a particular bathhouse was healthy for a particular body, at a particular time. By mapping out these complexities, the chapter brings attention to how different interpretative frameworks and practical circumstance interlinked in the day-to-day determination of what was healthy. While health was a signifier of the good life, it was also understood as situation-dependent, tied to body types and related to places.

Mary Lindemann has noted that 'the history of health in early modern society remains a story of the relationship of people to places.'[7] Yet, studies have often tended to focus on either places of health or the people frequenting them. Important work has been done on the understanding of

3 The Stockholm Bath Master's Guild received guild privileges in 1657. Flintberg, *Apothekares Badares och Chirurgers Förmoner.*

4 Carlsson, 'Om badstugor och bad'; Talve, 'Bastu och badstugor'; Talve, *Bastu och torkhus*; Troels-Lund, *Dagligt liv*, 316; Curman, *Om bad*; Skeri, *Renlighet och bekvämlighet.* Similar arguments have been made regarding late medieval European bathing cultures: see Vigarello, *Concepts of Cleanliness.* On socialising at the early modern spa, see, e.g., Herbert, 'Gender and the Spa.'

5 With the exception of references by historians of medicine to bath masters as agents at the medical marketplace. Lindberg, *Kirurgernas historia*; Fors, 'Medicine and the Making of a City.' See also Hjelt, *Svenska och finska medicinalverkets historia*, vols 1–2.

6 See the introduction to this volume: Forss and Eyice, 'Meanings of Health.'

7 Lindemann, *Medicine and Society*, 216.

the body in the early modern period, for example pointing out that the body was understood to be open to influences from the environment through a permeable skin.[8] However, research on the body has arguably in practice had a tendency to focus primarily on the body itself.[9] Conversely, health geographers have used concepts such as the idea of 'therapeutic places' to capture the cultural perception that some social spaces have been considered healthier than others.[10] Similarly, material history has looked at how, for example, 'the material conditions of the sickchamber substantially shaped the patient's sensations of sickness.'[11] Though valuable for bringing attention to how features such as architecture and material objects have been used to signify health, these approaches are less useful in capturing the nuances of how the early modern body was understood to be affected by immediate factors in the surrounding world, as well as by the actions and interactions between human bodies.

The present study instead focuses attention on conceptions of health articulated in relation to the *interplay* between places and bodies. I contend that the extent to which the bathhouse was understood as healthy was directly related to who used it and under what circumstances. Thus, the early modern Swedish sweat bath culture is used here as a case study that emphasises how conceptions of health were situated in relation to people's expectations of the character of certain places, and in relation to ideas about what happened to different bodies in those places.

The empirical analysis draws on a wide range of sources. To begin with, it relies on a survey of medical advice literature published in Sweden from the sixteenth century to the middle of the eighteenth century.[12] Many of these texts were printed as standalone publications, but medical advice was also incorporated into other genres, such as almanacs and treatises on *oeconomia* (Swe. *hushållningslitteratur, husfaderslitteratur*; Ger. *Hausväterliteratur*).[13] To

8 Runesson, *Blod, kött och tårar*; Roper, 'Martin Luther's Body'; Rublack, 'Fluxes'; Duden, *The Woman Beneath the Skin.*

9 Research on climate theory constitutes an obvious exception to this trend: Wear, 'Place, Health, and Disease'; Miller, '"Airs, Waters, and Places" in History.' Joanna Bourke's model for studying pain also constitutes a bridging of perspectives: Bourke, 'Pain: Metaphor, Body, and Culture'; Bourke, *The Story of Pain.*

10 See Gesler, 'Therapeutic Landscapes'; Bell et al., 'From Therapeutic Landscapes to Healthy Spaces'; Collins, *The Architecture and Landscape of Health.*

11 Newton, 'Inside the Sickchamber,' 530.

12 I have aimed to be as comprehensive as possible, including both widely circulated works and more marginal publications.

13 See Runefelt, *Hushållningens dygder*, ch. 4. Pocket-sized printed almanacs were exceedingly popular in early modern Europe. In Sweden, almanacs were imported from Germany, and from

gain insight into the experiences of individual bathers, the study examines travel narratives and diaries which refer to visits to bathhouses, and includes analyses of court records relating to crimes committed in, or in relation to, bathhouses. While these sources cannot be said to be representative of all early modern Swedish or Finnish bathers, they are valuable in showing modes of reasoning that were accepted, or on occasion rejected, by local communities and by the medical and juridical authorities.[14]

An examination of the Swedish sweat bath culture contributes to international debates on the history of health and bathing by highlighting the importance of paying attention to how European trends were localised and occurred at different times across the continent. Historians have long debated how practices of bathing related to cleanliness and health in early modern Europe. A dominant view has been that early modern people considered washing with water detrimental, instead changing their clothes as a means to maintain cleanliness. This view, however, has been challenged in recent years.[15] For instance, research on early modern England has demonstrated that washing and bathing was an essential part in numerous practices thought to help preserve existing good health, and to cure certain illnesses.[16] The Swedish sweat bath culture further challenges the view that bathing for health was broadly viewed with suspicion. However, in contrast to recent work on England, cleanliness does not play a significant role in the accounts of early modern Swedish bathhouses. Instead, as recent research has begun to explore, the connection between bathing and hygiene seems to have become more pronounced in the nineteenth and twentieth century in the Nordic region.[17]

While sweat baths were ubiquitous in Swedish cities and in the countryside throughout the sixteenth and seventeenth century, sweat bath practices changed in the eighteenth century and largely disappeared in

the late sixteenth century produced locally. Nordenmark argues that the Swedish almanacs were predominantly translations of German works. However, the fact that they were translated into Swedish meant that they were intended to be used by a Swedish audience, making them relevant to study for their part in shaping practices of health in Sweden. See Nordenmark, *Naturvetenskapernas historia*; Jensen, *Astrology*, 9. For the status of astrology in early modern Sweden, see Kjellgren, *Taming the Prophets*.

14 On the use of court records for historical analysis, see Toivo, 'Discerning Voices and Values.'

15 North, *Sweet and Clean?*; Vigarello, *Concepts of Cleanliness*; Van Bavel, 'The Economic Origins of Cleanliness.'

16 North, *Sweet and Clean?*; Smith, *Clean*.

17 Annola, Drakman, and Ulväng, eds., *Med tvål, vatten och flit*; Wiell, *Bad mot Lort och Sjukdom*. Note, however, that one possibility here is that 'clean' (Swe. *ren*) was understood to be part of the concept of health. See *Swedish Academy Dictionary* (*SAOB*), 'ren adj.'

parts of southern and western Sweden.[18] Focusing on the earlier part of the period, the current study does not discuss these changes in bathing in detail – they warrant a separate study.[19] Similarly, there were geographical difference regarding bathing culture within the Swedish realm. These differences have been studied in some detail by folklorist Illmar Talve, who notes that sweat baths continued to be common in the north and east for a longer period than in the south and southwest.[20] Despite some differences, it is my contention that there were enough similarities that we can speak of a common sweat bath culture in early modern Sweden.[21] That said, I do comment on geographic differences and change over time where it has a bearing on the present analysis, and it is worth noting that cultural practices underwent change over the course of the period in question.

The chapter begins by outlining the material and social conditions that, I argue, made people associate the bathhouse with health. The second part of the analysis considers how medical writers understood a visit to the Swedish bathhouse to affect northern bodies in particular ways. The third section examines in more detail what people understood happened to a person's body when he or she entered the sweat bath. The analysis moves between the early modern understanding of the bathhouse as a place, and what people believed happened to bodies in that place, while paying attention to how the understanding of what was healthy was articulated in relation to these factors.

Health in the bathhouse

What did a visit to an early modern Swedish bathhouse entail, and what material and social features made people associate it with health? To begin with, it is worth noting that the seemingly straightforward word 'bathing' (Swe. *bada*) referred to several different activities. The Swedish clergyman Isac Erici, building on the German *oeconomia*-writer Johannes Colerus, stated that there were three kinds of bathing: sweating in a heated chamber, submerging oneself in a waterfilled bathtub, and sweating in a container that enclosed the body, though not the head.[22] In addition, the term 'bath'

18 Talve, 'Bastu och badstugor.' On the medieval bathing culture, see Carlsson, 'Om badstugor.'

19 I am addressing these processes of change in a coming publication.

20 Talve, 'Bastu och badstugor'; Talve, *Bastu och torkhus*. See also Strandberg, *Koppning i Finland*.

21 See also Nordström, *Nordiska bad*; Troels-Lund, *Dagligt liv*, 316.

22 Erici, *M. Joh. Coleri Oeconomia*, 181. Harpesträng describes bathing in a heated container, see Harpesträng, 'Här byrias läkedombir,' 6. See also Elfving, *Kort anledning*, 12–14.

could also refer to the application of a wet bandage, and to submersion in a pool, sea, or lake.[23] The focal point of the present study is the sweat bath, partly because that particular form of bathing was widespread in early modern Sweden, and partly because it was seen by contemporaries as something peculiar to this part of the world.[24] As discussed in some detail below, the heat and humidity of the bath was understood to induce sweating, which would cause the body to excrete harmful or superfluous elements, and thereby also affect a person's humoral balance. Depending on the status of the body prior to sweating, the bath would lead to better or worse health.[25] Thus, a visit to a sweat bath was understood to have health effects regardless of whether a person made the visit with the intention of undergoing medical treatment.

The design of the bathhouse and types of bathing varied between different parts of Sweden, between city and countryside, and between bathhouses intended for the rich and for the poor.[26] However, some general characteristics can also be seen. A sweat bath was prepared in a separate house or chamber: this was the bathhouse. The Swedish word for bathhouse, *badstuga*, much like the Finnish equivalent *sauna*, referred both to the building and to the sweat bath itself.[27] Larger establishments had a room for undressing attached to the heated chamber, though this does not seem to have been standard everywhere.[28] The room itself was heated through a stove made of stones or bricks.[29]

In addition to the rituals of the sweat bath, bathers could engage in other health practices in the bathhouse. One example of this was cupping therapy, a form of bloodletting effected with minor cuts to the skin and the application of cups or horns that drew out blood, aiming at restoring the

23 E.g., Anonymous, 'Ett Bad för Hiertats Swaghet.'

24 Sweat baths could be dry or wet through steam. Moreover, the smoke from the stove could be diverted through a chimney, or, as common in Finland, filling the room. However, the discussions about the health effects of the baths seldom made distinctions between different kinds of sweat baths.

25 On the medical significance of sweat in the early modern period, see Stolberg, 'Sweat'; van Gent, *Magic, Body and Self*, 94.

26 Talve describes differences in building style in some detail: Talve, *Bastu och torkhus.*

27 *SAOB*, 'badstuga.' Several different spellings appear in the sources, e.g., 'bastuwa,' 'badhestuffwa.' Another term used is 'swettstuga' (Eng. 'sweat house'). See, *SAOB*, 'svettstuga.' In Finnish, the corresponding term is *sauna.* I use the terms bathhouse, sauna, and sweat bath interchangeably. In addition, I point out when the historical accounts are vague about what kind of bathing they refer to.

28 As seen in Stenberg's comments about Finns walking naked out of the sauna. Stenberg, *Pehr Stenbergs levernesbeskrivning*, 1:237.

29 See Talve, *Bastu och torkhus*, 69.

humoral balance of the afflicted body.[30] The association between cupping therapy and the sweat bath is seen, for example, in early modern almanacs that used the symbol for a cupping device to indicate on what days it would be beneficial to bathe as well as undergo a cupping therapy (see Figure 3.1).[31] Hindrik Strandberg notes, regarding a somewhat later period, that other bloodletting therapies were commonly performed in Finland in saunas.[32] There is also evidence that rural communities used bathhouses as sickrooms, bringing ill persons to the bathhouse and keeping them there for extended periods of time.[33] Thus, a set of different kinds of health practices were linked to the bathhouse, in addition to the sweat bath itself.

In Stockholm, this was even more pronounced in that the masters of the Bathing Guild were granted privileges in 1657 to treat minor wounds and cut hair, in addition to run the city's major public bathhouses.[34] The accreditation of the bath masters was contested by the city's barber surgeons, indicating that the medical status of the bath masters did not stand unchallenged.[35] However, when the medical physicians of the Collegium Medicum received their instructions in 1663, the bath masters were one of the groups the collegium was tasked with overseeing.[36] Though the bath masters did not undergo a long-term professionalisation similar to medical doctors or barber surgeons – discussed in Hjalmar Fors's and Maria Sjöberg's chapters in this volume – it seems clear that the bath masters were considered to be part of the medical marketplace of Stockholm in the seventeenth century.[37] It is likely that this was one further factor that made people perceive the bathhouse as an establishment that promoted good health.

While most bathers did not comment on what it felt like to take a sweat bath, we have some indications that it was an experience that was

30 Cupping therapies can also be bloodless, or dry, though Strandberg notes that therapies that drew blood seem to have been more common in both Sweden and Finland. Strandberg, *Koppning i Finland*, 54–56.

31 Strandberg, *Koppning i Finland*, 27.

32 Strandberg, *Koppning i Finland*, 18.

33 *Gender and Work* (*GaW*), case no. 9290; Landsarkivet i Vadstena, Göta Hovrätts arkiv, Advokatfiskalens arkiv, Från underrätterna inkomna renovationer … Kronobergs län, 1650–1651, 10 January 1651; Landsarkivet i Östersund, Jämtlands domsagas häradsrätts arkiv, vol. A I: 15a, 27, 28, 29, and 30 November 1694.

34 Flintberg, *Apothekares Badares och Chirurgers Förmoner*; *Stockholms stads ordinantier*, 131.

35 See Lindberg, *Kirurgernas historia*.

36 Hjelt, *Svenska och finska medicinalverkets historia*, 1:10–12.

37 I examine the activities of the Bathing Guild in relation to knowledge production in a forthcoming article.

understood in terms of bodily pain and pleasure.[38] For example, to Guiseppe Acerbi, an Italian traveller who visited saunas in Finland at the end of the eighteenth century, the experience of entering the sweat bath was one of bodily discomfort and even pain, contrasted with the ease with which the Finns endured the bath. Acrebi describes that when entering the sauna 'I could not breathe, and in the space of a minute at most, I verily believe, must have been suffocated.'[39] For most baths, we do not know how hot the temperature was, though some early measurements from the eighteenth century indicate temperatures ranging from 45°C to 75°C.[40] This perhaps does not sound so excessive, yet it is clear that it was experienced as such by Acerbi, who regarded a bath of 70°C to be unbearable.

Furthermore, Acerbi's sensations were acerbated by the contrast he perceived between himself and the easy experience of the locals who enjoyed the heat. He wrote in his travel account that: 'My astonishment was so great that I could scarcely believe my senses, when I found that those people remain together, and amuse themselves for the space of half an hour, and sometimes an whole hour [in the sauna].'[41] We see here how Acerbi experienced the sweat bath through overpowering bodily sensations, but also in relation to his fellow bathers. This is a point that aligns well with historian Joanna Bourke's argument that the sensation of pain should be seen as experienced both through the body, through language, and through culture.[42] Bearing this in mind, the fact that the bathhouse was a place where people went to socialise is significant for the experience of the bath having a good or bad effect on a person's health.

The bath itself entailed several semi-ritualised steps that were dependent on the interaction between bathers. While part of the bathing ritual consisted of the bather sitting or lying down in the heated chamber, other elements required assistance either from a bathhouse attendant or from a fellow bather. According to a Frenchman who visited Stockholm in the mid seventeenth century, part of the sweat bath consisted of a female bathing attendant taking his arms and scrubbing

> first one and then the other with soap and horsehair brush, and then [she] scrubs the body from top to toe, except for that part (you know

38 E.g., Ödmann, *Hågkomster från Hembygden*, 21; Anonymous [French traveller]. *Den franske kammartjänarens resa,* 161.

39 Acerbi, *Travels through Sweden*, 298.

40 The lower temperatures referred to wet steam baths and the higher to dry baths. Acerbi, *Travels through Sweden*, 298; Rolandsson, 'Physiologiska Rön och Anmärkningar,' 70–71.

41 Acerbi, *Travels through Sweden*, 298.

42 Bourke, 'Pain: Metaphor, Body, and Culture.'

> what I mean) which one washes oneself. And then when one is completely white from lather, one rises and she pours a bucket of lukewarm water over the head, which completely removes the lather. This is repeated two or three times.[43]

At a public establishment like the one described in the Frenchman's account, an employee of the bathhouse performed the washing, while in a bathhouse belonging to, for instance, a farm, members of the household would have washed each other.[44] Regardless, the ritual practices associated with the bath meant that the bathers were directly involved in each other's bodily experiences of bathing.

It has been noted that elsewhere in Europe the intimate interaction between the sexes in bathhouses led to moral anxiety and to concern over the spread of disease.[45] For instance, public bathhouses were closed in the early fifteenth century because they became associated with the rapidly spreading syphilis epidemic. Contemporary observers connected the spread of this disease with immoral behaviour, and in particular, with prostitution.[46] As seen in the introduction to the present volume, health could also contain connotations to virtue in early modern Swedish public discourse. However, while foreign visitors to Scandinavia certainly seem to have perceived a visit to the bathhouse as sexually charged, the medical advice literature – including advice on syphilis – from sixteenth- and seventeenth-century Sweden did not condemn the public bathhouses as unhealthy in connection with endangering a person's virtue.[47] There were some suggestions that bathing should be restricted during outbreaks of the plague – an illness that did have moral overtones in early modern discourse – in Sweden.[48] For example, the bishop and scholar Laurentius Paulinus Gothus suggested in 1623 that public bathhouses should be closed during plague outbreaks.[49] However, comments in the Swedish advice literature about restricting bathing during plague outbreaks seems to have stemmed more from concern about contagion

43 Anonymous [French traveller]. *Den franske kammartjänarens resa*, 160–161.

44 This, however, did not exclude social hierarchies in who washed whom. See for example *GaW*, case no. 5387; Acerbi, *Travels through Sweden*, 338–339.

45 Carlsson, 'Bad och Badstugor,' 139. Similarly, the intimacy of the *hammam* caused concern about morals in eighteenth-century Aleppo. See Semerdjian, 'Naked Anxiety.'

46 Smith, *Clean*, 180–181; Lindberg, *Kirurgernas historia*, 35.

47 Forss, 'Some Like It Hot.'

48 Healy, 'Why Me? Why Now? How?'; Lemnius, *Emoot pestilentzie*, 9r; Petri, *Then swenska kyrkeordningen*, xciii.

49 Paulinus Gothus, *Loimoscopia*, 101r.

transmission through bad air – *miasma* – than about issues of morality.[50] That is not to say that bathhouses were not used for illicit sexual affairs in early modern Sweden. On the contrary, it is clear that they were at times.[51] However, it seems that the bathhouse was not generally considered to be a place of immorality to an extent that it diminished its status as a place of health.

In sum, I have suggested here that there were a number of features of the sweat bath culture that, to the early modern observer, associated it with health. First, the material conditions of the bath, its heat and humidity, were understood to affect a person's health through sweating. Second, people visited the bathhouse to receive other health therapies, in addition to sweating. Third, and building on Bourke, I suggest that the social interaction during the sweat bath intensified the experience that the bath affected a person's body. It is not possible to say conclusively if people visited the bathhouse because they conceived of it as a place that promoted good health, or if it became a place associated with health practices because it was used as a sickroom and as a basis for the activities of the bath masters, who were considered as healers in relation to other treatments they performed. Likely, the different features of the sweat bath culture reinforced each other, making it a place understood to affect health.

The northern body takes a sweat bath

To what extent did early modern writers conceive of the sweat bath as a feature of local society and climate, and what role did conceptions of health play in these discussions? To answer this question, let us first turn to Olaus Magnus, the scholar and last Catholic archbishop of Sweden who detailed the mores of the Swedes in his *Historia de Gentibus Septentrionalibus* (History of the northern people), published in 1555. Describing the local sweat bath culture, Olaus Magnus claimed that the cold weather in Sweden made it necessary for people to visit bathhouses. He noted that although people in all parts of the world practised bathing, '[n]owhere in the world is their use as necessary as it is in the northern countries.' The sulphurous baths that were common in other localities could not cure 'the common illnesses of this country' and instead people resorted to their own kinds of bathhouses.[52]

50 On plague and miasma, see Healy, 'Why Me? Why Now? How?,' 45.

51 See for example *GaW*, case no. 5387.

52 Magnus, *Historia om de nordiska folken*, book XV, ch. 35.

In this account, Olaus Magnus makes a direct connection between the cold climate of Sweden, the nature of local illnesses, and people's health requirements.

Olaus Magnus's argument draws on the Hippocratic treatise *On Airs, Waters, and Places*, which was influential in the early modern period, and according to which places and their respective weather conditions were understood to bear a direct relationship to health.[53] For example, the inhabitants of towns facing north, and thus receiving an excess of cold and dry wind, were believed to suffer more from dry coughs and other lung diseases, while those living in towns facing south were prone to dysentery.[54] In a related discourse, the earth was understood to be divided into zones, or *climata*, with conditions that influenced human characteristics such as height and mental faculties. For example, the northern temperate zone, which encompassed most of the European latitudes, was believed to foster tall, quick-tempered individuals. In contrast, the frigid zones around the poles were understood to be uninhabitable, or at least detrimental to human health.[55]

For early modern Swedish scholars, these theories posed a problem. The notion that Sweden's inhabitants were slow witted and outwardly less handsome than their neighbours further south held little appeal. Instead, Swedish commentators attempted to find ways around the standard environmentalist narrative of physiology. Thus, in his 1578 advice book about common ailments, the medical doctor Benedictus Olai argued that, in fact, 'in these Northerly lands people have stronger constitutions,' rather than the expected weaker constitutions of the far north.[56] The reason for this resilience was that the populace had been hardened by the harsh weather. Thus, Olai used the standard proposition of climate theory (that climate affected physiology), yet adjusted it so that it presented Swedes in a more positive light.

Olai supported his argument through the example of the sweat bath: Swedes could tolerate the heat of the sweat bath better than people from other places. The sweat bath was less harmful for people from the north than it could be for others, partly because of the strong constitutions of the people from Sweden, and partly because they had 'become used to sweat baths through upbringing.' Nature and nurture alike had made the

53 Wear, 'Place, Health, and Disease'; Miller, '"Airs, Waters, and Places" in History.'

54 Miller, '"Airs, Waters, and Places" in History.'

55 On the relationship between ideas about weather and the theory of climatic zones, see Miglietti, 'Climate Theory: An "Invented Tradition"?.'

56 Olai, *Een Nyttigh Läkere Book*, 1r–2v.

Swedes well suited for the sweat bath. The result, as Olai saw it, was that the Swedes required medical advice from someone who 'has knowledge about all circumstances that, in addition to medical knowledge, should be known and heeded,' that is, a person who knew local culture.[57] The bodily constitutions of the people in Sweden, shaped by climate and habits, required localised medical expertise.

While not all medical authors used the example of the sweat bath to make their case, the idea that medical knowledge had to relate to local conditions was repeated in publications throughout the early modern period.[58] For example, the medical doctor Johan Hartmann from Turku (in Finland) noted in the 1756 introduction to his medical book, which was aimed at the general public, that he had amended the advice so that everyone would understand it, and that he had 'corrected and adjusted [the advice] to our Nordic climate.'[59]

Authors like Hartmann and Olai probably wrote out of medicinal convictions, but it is also worth noting that their localised presentation of climate theory gave them another reason why people should read their books, rather than consult medical treatises from abroad. Andrew Wear points to a similar case where early modern English writers promoting colonisation in America used Hippocratic theories to emphasise that the weather in the New World would suit 'our English bodyes.'[60] In both cases, climate theory was reinterpreted and used to endorse a certain agenda. As I have explored in previous studies, similar motifs can be seen in early modern works in geography and travel writing.[61] However, in the context of medical advice books, the claim that local knowledge was needed had the further effect of advancing an understanding of health as linked to specific places, and of health as connected to the adaptability of bodily constitutions.

There is a recurring theme in these comments that sweat baths are healthier for persons who make it a habit to visit the bathhouse. A French seventeenth-century visitor to Stockholm claimed that 'since the cold in this country is so severe, there are bathhouses where people go to sweat whenever they want to.'[62] Writers emphasised – in line with Hippocratic

57 Olai, *Een Nyttigh Läkere Book*, 1r–2v.

58 See for example, Berchelt, *Om pestilentzien*, 3r; Lindh, *Huusz-apoteek*, 3v–4r; Lemnius, *Emoot pestilentzie*, 1v, 4v; Erici, *M.Joh. Coleri Oeconomia*, 2r, 124, 125.

59 Haartman, *Tydelig underrättelse*, 14.

60 Wear, 'Place, Health, and Disease,' 452. See also Ordahl Kupperman, 'The Puzzle of the American Climate.'

61 Forss, *The Old, the New and the Unknown*, 111–114.

62 Anonymous [French traveller], *Den Franske kammartjänarens resa*, 161.

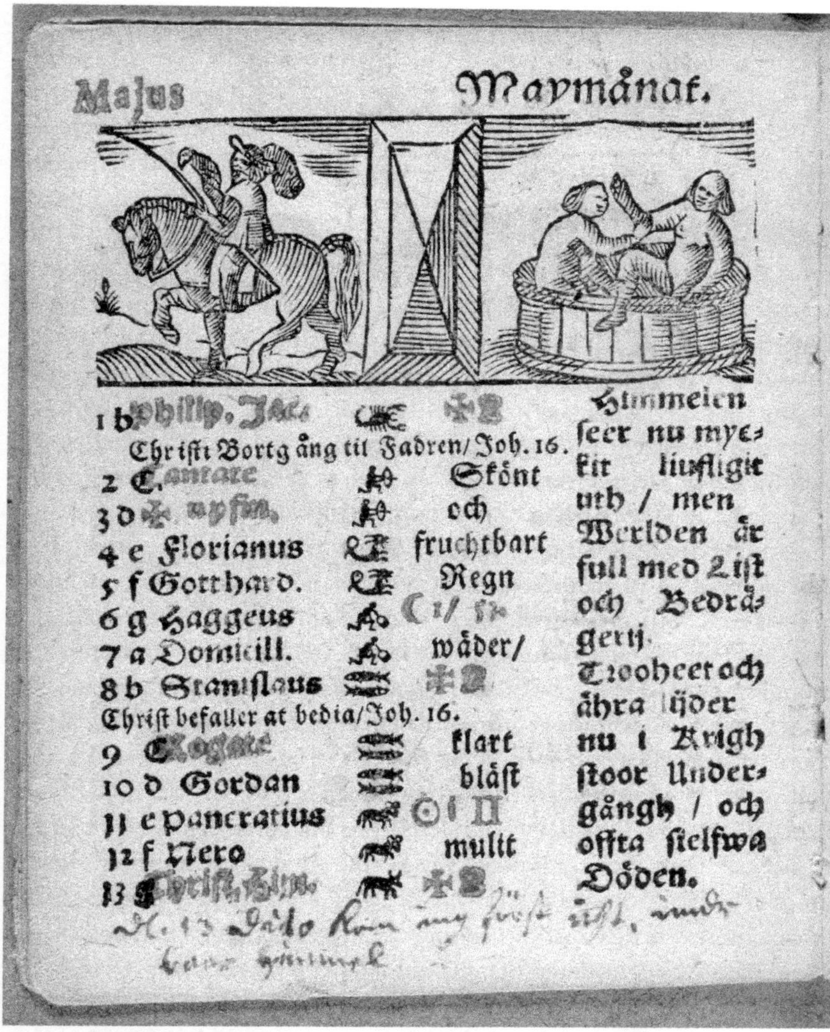
Majus Maymånat.
1 b Philip. Jac.
Christi Bortgång til Fadren/Joh. 16.
2 c Cantate Skönt
3 d och
4 e Florianus fruchtbart
5 f Gotthard. Regn
6 g Haggeus
7 a Domicill. wåder/
8 b Stanislaus
Christ befaller at bedia/Joh. 16.
9 c Rogate klart
10 d Gordian blåst
11 e Pancratius
12 f Nereo mulit
13 g Christi Him.
Himmelen seer nu myckit liufligit uth / men Werlden är full med List och Bedrägerij. Troheet och åhra lijder nu i Krigh stoor Undergångh / och offta sielfwa Döden.

Figure 3.1. Almanac for May 1675. Two bathers represent the Zodiac sign Gemini. The almanac advises bathing on 1, 8, and 13 May. Stephanus Fuhrman, *Almanach, På thet Åhret effter wårs Herres Jesu Christi Nåde rijke Födelse 1675* (Stockholm, [1674]). Image: David Frederiksen, Royal Library, Stockholm.

dietary advice – that health was linked to what people were used to.[63] Sweat baths were common in early modern Sweden; hence Swedish bodies could stand the heat of the sweat bath better than people from other places. Frequenting sweat baths changed a person's bodily constitution, and health

63 The Hippocratic corpus also advised bathing to maintain health. See Dvorjetski, *Leisure, Pleasure and Healing*, 84.

advice needed to be adjusted accordingly. In this reasoning, health was, in a somewhat circular argument, directly related to the activities people engaged in.

The connection between cold weather and sweat baths was also expressed in advice about when to bathe, found in printed almanacs and in treatises on *oeconomia*. Recommendations and educational rhymes in the margins of the almanacs proposed ideal times for bathing, as in a 1622 almanac, which noted that 'In April, the body will be cleansed from all evil moisture that he has gathered all through the winter. Thus, it is healthy to bathe, sweat, purge, [and] let blood on all parts of the body, excepting the neck and throat.'[64] This advice was similarly expressed in a treatise on *oeconomia*, the author noting that it was advisable to bathe in springtime because 'the sweat pores are closed by the cold' during winter.[65] A vignette of the Zodiac sign Gemini showed as two persons in a bath tub next to the month of May (see Figure 3.1), further associated spring time with bathing.[66] We see here how the human body was understood as porous, affected by the surrounding environment – both in immediate terms in relation to the hot micro-climate of the sweat bath, and in relation to the cold of the northern latitudes.[67]

In all of the examples discussed here, a cold and harsh climate is presented as an established feature of a rather vaguely defined 'north.' People seem to have visited bathhouses also during the warmer summer months yet there was clearly a perception that the cold climate itself created a need for the heat of the sweat bath. A perception of the cold of 'the north' being in some regards unhealthy contributed to the conceptualisation of the bathhouse as a place that was healthy. Yet the effect of the northern climate on physiology was not the only factor to take into consideration, as the advice literature also draws a connection between habits and health: the sweat bath was considered beneficial for a person who was used to it, but potentially dangerous for a person who was not. What thus emerges is an assumption that longstanding habits and environmental factors alike affect

64 [Herlicius, *Almanac for 1622*]. The title page of the copy of the almanac that I have consulted, kept at the Royal Library in Stockholm, is missing. G. E. Klemming and G. Eneström's survey of early modern Swedish almanacs mention two almanacs printed for the year 1622, one by Herlicius and one by Forsius, and this is not Forsius's almanac. Klemming and G. Eneström, *Svenska almanachor*, 5.

65 Erici, *M. Joh. Coleri Oeconomia*, 182. See also Forsius, *Almanah …* [*1609*]; [Herlicius, *Almanach for 1622*].

66 Quensel, *Almanach På Åhret … 1724*; Fuhrman, *Almanach … 1675*; Fuhrman, *Almanach … 1676*.

67 Wear, 'Place, Health, and Disease'; Miller, '"Airs, Waters, and Places" in History'; Stolberg, 'Sweat,' 515. On this paradigm in a Swedish context, see Drakman, *När kroppen slöt sig*.

human physiology, and that both factors have worked together to make the sweat bath healthier for Swedish bodies than for those from other parts of the world.

Bathing to cure illness and to preserve health

What did people believe happened to their bodies when they entered a sweat bath? As noted already, the main health effect attributed to the sweat bath was sweating. On the one hand, sweating was understood to cure certain ailments by restoring the humoral balance and ridding the body of excess fluids. On the other hand, and in accordance with Hippocratic theory, sweating was understood as part of a set of activities – the six *nonnaturals* – that people should engage in as a means to maintain an already existing level of well-being. The French mid-seventeenth century visitor to Stockholm, referred to earlier, highlighted this dual effect in his description of Swedish bathing habits, noting that 'there is no rheumatism that cannot be cured by it, and they [the Swedes] say that it keeps them from falling ill.'[68] Bathing was thus an activity that could both cure illness and preserve health.

That said, advice books often contradicted each other about what a sweat bath could cure and in what situations it was dangerous to bathe. Medical authors suggested that sweat baths were a remedy for ailments as diverse as colic, melancholy, wrath, pain in the limbs, rashes, and certain fevers, to name just a few.[69] However, they all agreed that the point of different kinds of baths was to allow trapped fluids to leave the body through sweating, thereby restoring the humoral balance.[70] This naturally also meant that there were many circumstances when taking a sweat bath could be detrimental to health by further exacerbating existing imbalances.[71]

The important guiding principle for advice on bathing was the understanding that a host of factors influenced the makeup of a person's physiology, and that what was good for one could be dangerous to another.[72] For example, the medical doctor Petrus Elfving, who in 1716 published an officially sanctioned medical advice book aimed at the general public, noted that different kinds of bathing, including sweat baths, constituted one of the

68 Anonymous [French traveller], *Den Franske kammartjänarens resa*, 161.

69 Haartman, *Tydelig underrättelse*, 93, 362; Broocman, *En Fulständig Swensk Hus-Hålds-Bok*, 236; Lindh, *Huusz-apoteek*, 89; Anonymous, 'Läkebok nr 3 Codex Huss,' 72.

70 E.g., Gothus, *Loimoscopia*, 80r.

71 E.g., Erici, *M.Joh. Coleri Oeconomia*, 182; Lindh, *Huusz-apoteek*, 153.

72 Haartman, *Tydelig underrättelse*, 21, 116; Erici, *M.Joh. Coleri Oeconomia*, 181–183.

methods available to treating symptoms of illness.[73] Yet, after giving this initial stamp of approval, Elfving was careful to expound on the situations and body types which should be considered before using different kinds of baths. He noted in particular that 'those who are unused to baths,' those with an excess of blood, or who are feverish, often find that bathing does not agree with them.[74] In the comment that people unused to bathing should be particularly careful we see again the idea that health was connected to a person's habits, and that habits could affect physiology.

According to humoral pathology, a person's complexion – that is, the composition of humours in the body – changed over the course of a lifetime from warmer and wetter to drier and colder.[75] This needed to be taken into account when considering if it would be good to take a bath. Swedish language almanacs from the first half of the seventeenth century often noted not only on what days it was particularly beneficial, from an astrological standpoint, to take a bath, but also whether the advice was directed at persons with sanguine, choleric, melancholy, or phlegmatic complexions.[76] Thus, David Herlicius, a medical doctor based in Stargard in Pomerania (in present day Poland), and whose almanacs were popular in Sweden in the early seventeenth century, advised that on Saturday 14 January 1632, it would be particularly good for young persons who had a choleric temperament to take a bath.[77] The basis for this advice was astrological observations about the position of the moon in relation to the zodiac signs, and underpinning these remarks was the supposition that the planets would affect the physical world – including the four humours and through them the human body – just as the moon affected the tide.[78] Important here is also the idea of the porosity of the human body, positing that the body could be influenced by larger environmental forces as well as by the bath itself.

That sweat baths could be considered more or less healthy at different points in a person's life is seen in the journal of the schoolteacher Petrus Magnus Gyllenius from Värmland in western Sweden. As a student in Turku in 1649, Gyllenius noted that he had visited a bathhouse, of which he wrote:

73 Elfving, *Kort anledning för en huushållare*, 12. The publication was supported by the *Collegium Medicum*.

74 Elfving, *Kort anledning för en huushållare*, 13.

75 Moreau, 'Complexion.'

76 E.g., Forsius, *Almanach ... [1608]*; Herlicius, *Calendarium*; Kexlerus, *Almanach*; Schomerus, *Almanach*.

77 Herlicius, *Almanach ... 1632*.

78 Jensen, *Astrology*, 20; Wallis, 'Medicine in Medieval Calendar Manuscripts'; Kjellgren, *Taming the Prophets*, 37. See, e.g., Fuhrman, *Almanach ... 1661*; Spole, *Almanach ... 1692*.

'I fell very ill from it, and was weak in my whole body for eight days before I was returned to health.'[79] However, later in life, Gyllenius took up bathing as a regular habit to treat the pain he suffered from in his limbs. While a visit to a bathhouse had made him ill in his youth, it was a habit he practised later in life with good health effects.

That the advice about bathing needed to be adjusted to body types and specific situations is further evidenced by how medical advice books described the relationship between bathhouses and the plague. In his 1623 treatise on the plague and its divine as well as natural aspects, Paulinus Gothus emphasised that sweating was an important protective bodily function against the plague, as well as a treatment for those afflicted by this illness, yet, as noted above, he also advised moderation with regards to sweat baths during plague outbreaks. In fact, healthy persons ought not 'to take baths often, only once a month' during outbreaks.[80] For the sick, Paulinius Gothus advised other, milder, remedies to promote sweating, such as drinking sweat-inducing concoctions, or covering the sick person with blankets and putting hot stones or heated water bottles in their beds. In all of his advice, he emphasised the importance of moderation – a notion that was central to Galenic/Hippocratic medicine and the health regimens centred around the theory of the six nonnaturals.

As noted already, Paulinus Gothus's understanding of bad air, so-called *miasma*, as a conduit for illness made him suggest that public venues, including bathhouses, should be closed during outbreaks of the plague so that the bad air would not spread through the public bathhouse. Paulinus Gothus made a distinction here between the unhealthy air of a public bathhouse and the potentially beneficial effects of taking a mild bath to induce sweating. This passage highlights that there were aspects of a bathhouse that could make people consider it both healthy and unhealthy, and it is an interesting point in relation to the idea of 'therapeutic places' explored by health geographers. For instance, Paulinus Gothus portrayed the bathhouse as both a therapeutic and untherapeutic place, indicating that the argument that a place was considered therapeutic in the early modern period needs to take into account the variability of factors that were understood to interact in the attribution of health.

Did people heed medical advice about how to determine if taking a bath was healthy? This is a difficult question to answer since there seldom is any evidence of a person choosing not to take a bath. We have seen that

79 Gyllenius, *Diarium Gylleanium*, 160.
80 Paulinus Gothus, *Loimoscopia*, 81r.

Petrus Magnus Gyllenius connected the activity of bathing with his health status (both in negative and positive ways) and that bathhouses could be used as sickrooms.[81] The case of an unexplained death in Stockholm gives some indication that following medical advice in practice might be more complicated still. The episode concerns the death of the boatswain Erik Simonson, who was found dead on a street one morning in August 1710. People in the neighbourhood told the court that Simonson had looked 'very ill,' and that he had 'come to Wife Annika and asked to use the bathhouse, but he had soon left, and the following morning they had found him lying dead in the street.'[82] Another set of witnesses reported that Simonson's wife had died a few days earlier from the same illness, and they also mentioned that Simonson had intended to go to the barber for bloodletting, but that he had not made it all the way.[83] As it turned out, Erik Simonson and his wife were two of the first victims of the last outbreak of the plague in Stockholm. It is unlikely that Simonson had known what illness he suffered from, or that he was aware that Paulinus Gothus, close to ninety years earlier, had advised those afflicted by the plague against visiting a bathhouse. The medical advice literature set out an understanding of the cause and effect of health and illness, yet it is hardly likely that all nuances of this translated into the health practices of the general populace.

Still, the witnesses and the court scribe who reported on Erik Simonson's death felt it relevant to mention the sweat bath in the court protocol. More to the point, the reports brought up Simonson's wish to take a sweat bath and to see the barber for bloodletting as part of the description of his illness. Simonson's last actions before he died indicated that he was indeed ill. For the court, this was important since they were investigating an unexplained death. At the start of the investigation, they had to contend with the possibility that Simonson could have been murdered. The evidence that he, during the last hours of his life, had behaved as an ill person – that is, he had wanted to take a sweat bath and to be bled – contributed to determining the cause of death. This indicates a shared understanding of the bathhouse as a place of health among the officials, Simonson, and the witnesses that were called in the case, beyond the complexities of when a particular bath would be considered healthy for a particular body type.

81 See also *GaW*, case no. 9290.

82 Stockholms stadsarkiv (SSA): Södra förstadens kämnärsrätt. Protokoll och domar i kriminalmål huvudserie: A3a Vol. 2, 1710, 814. I am grateful to Karin Sennefelt for bringing this case to my attention.

83 SSA: Södra förstadens kämnärsrätt. Protokoll och domar i kriminalmål huvudserie, A3a vol. 2, 1710, 817.

Over time, the medical authorities in Stockholm expressed increasing concern about the health effects of bathing among the lower classes. While medical advice literature still described sweat baths as beneficial, if not too hot and when used in moderation, there seems to have occurred a slow change in the eighteenth century where the understanding of the bathhouse as a place of health became contested among the elite. For instance, the Collegium Medicum published a pamphlet in 1755, condemning the practice among Finnish mothers of taking their newborn babies into the bathhouse.[84] In the mid-eighteenth century, the sweat bath culture was changing, and becoming a less common activity among the upper echelons of society in Stockholm.[85] Michael Stolberg has pointed to a similar trend in eighteenth-century Europe more generally, where sweating as a curative method came under increasing suspicion from the medical authorities, in opposition to lay practice.[86] It seems that when the role of the bathhouse in society changed, the perception of the bathhouse as a place conducive to health also changed.

Conclusions

This study has argued that the sweat baths in early modern Sweden were understood as places that affected health. A person's illness or health was confirmed through their actions. In early modern Sweden, one such action was visiting a sweat bath. This supposition is borne out in the early modern medical advice literature, and in evidence from ego-documents and court records.

The sweat bath was thought to possess certain material conditions that could affect a person's health. The health effects of the sweat bath were not, however, understood as fixed. Instead, the characteristics of the bath were interpreted directly in relation to conceptions of the humoral body. An examination of the bathhouse in early modern Swedish society thus brings attention to the intricate link between conceptions of the physical environment and a person's body in early modern conceptions of health.

While mirroring themes discussed throughout this book, the present focus on the body in the bathhouse also draws attention to a more situation-dependent evaluation of health. While the bathhouse was associated with health practices through its material conditions, the professional groups active in the bathhouse, and the variety of activities commonly performed

84 Wolff, *Späda Barns Nödiga ans.*
85 Talve, *Bastu och Torkhus.*
86 Stolberg, 'Sweat,' 516.

there, the effect of a sweat bath on a particular body was not healthy by default. In the bathhouse, health was dependent on the humoral composition of the person who was bathing – which in turn was understood as shaped by factors such as the natural environment, astrological forces, the bathing person's habits over the course of a lifetime – and, as seen in the case of Guiseppe Acerbi, interpreted in relation to the experiences of the other bathers. The body does not feel in isolation, and the fact that the bathhouse was a place of socialising likely affected experiences of health in this particular environment. Taken together, the interplay between this rather large set factors shaped what health was understood to be for a particular body in a particular bathhouse.

Yet little or no instruction was given in the medical advice literature about what factors were more important to consider when determining if a sweat bath would affect a person's health in a positive or negative way, or on how to maintain balance between contradicting advice. Although the medical literature often claimed that it was directed to the general public, it is likely that these descriptions also sought to convey the need for the expert medical advice that their authors embodied.

This makes it relevant to ask: How widespread was the understanding that a visit to the bathhouse could heal a sick body in early modern Sweden? While it is not possible to make quantitative assessments of the prevalence of the understanding that the bathhouse affected health, the references to bathing as evidence of illness brought up in a variety of different kinds of sources indicate that we are looking at a common understanding. The fact that the bath could be used in a court case as evidence indicating a person's diminished health goes some way to support the view that sweat baths were a known and accepted mode of healing. It is also worth noting that the sources analysed in this study come from different geographical locations in early modern Sweden, and they cover a period from the late sixteenth century to the mid-eighteenth century. While the material does not say anything about how often bathing was used for healing among the populace, it does indicate that through the better part of the early modern period, sweat baths were accepted by medical practitioners, local communities, city dwellers, and the authorities in Sweden as places for treating the ill.

Although considered potentially health promoting, the bathhouse was also at times considered to be detrimental to health. For instance, implied in the advice that some days were good for bathing is an understanding that to bathe on other days was unwise. Similarly, the comment that sweat baths were less dangerous to the Swedes who were used to them indicates that taking a sweat bath was potentially unhealthy to others.

That said, the different kinds of materials analysed here consistently indicate that taking a sweat bath was understood to affect the body. Some effects were temporary – like sweating while in the sauna – and others were understood to cause permanent changes, like the body becoming habituated to the sauna from frequent bathing. However, taking a sweat bath would always have some effect on your body, and, moreover, these effects were conceptualised in terms of health. The effects on the body of a sweat bath were not neutral, but instead were framed as either good or bad for a person's well-being. This is particularly interesting since, as suggested in this study, people did not only bathe for health reasons. Socialising could be a reason to take a sweat bath in early modern Sweden, but the act of bathing would still affect a person's health.

Bibliography

Archival sources

Landsarkivet i Vadstena,
Göta Hovrätts arkiv, Advokatfiskalens arkiv.

Landsarkivet i Östersund
Jämtlands domsagas häradsrätts arkiv.

Stockholms stadsarkiv (SSA)
Södra förstadens kämnärsrätt.

Printed works

Acerbi, Giuseppe. *Travels through Sweden, Finland, and Lapland, to the North Cape, in the years 1798 and 1799*, vol. 1. London: Printed for J. Mawman, 1802.

Anonymous, 'Ett Bad för Hiertats Swaghet.' In Conrad Quensel, *Almanach På Åhret efter Jesu Christi Nåderijka Födelse 1724*. Stockholm, 1723.

Anonymous [French traveller]. *Den franske kammartjänarens resa: Minnen från länderna i norr på 1660-talet*, translated by Mari Bacquin and edited by Ingemar Oscarsson. Stockholm: Atlantis, 2013.

Anonymous, 'Läkebok nr 3 Codex Huss.' In *Läke- och örteböcker från Sveriges medeltid, första häftet*, edited by G. E. Klemming. Samlingar utg. Af Svenska Fornskrift-Sällskapet, del 26. Stockholm: Kongl. Boktryckeriet, 1883.

Berchelt, Simon. *Om pestilentzien och hennes orsaker, och huru man kan weta, om wädhret är aff pestilentzien förgifftet, och om een är siuk, om thet är pestilentzie eller icke*. Stockholm, 1589.

Broocman, Reinerus Reineri. *En Fulständih Swensk Hus-Hålds-Bok*, edited by Håkan Tunón. Stockholm and Uppsala: Kungl. Skogs- och Lantbruksakademien and Centrum för biologisk mångfald, 2016.

Elfving, Peter. *Kort anledning för en huushållare på landzbygden wid påkommande sjukdomar*. Stockholm, 1716.

Erici, Isac. *M. Joh. Coleri Oeconomia, Thet är Hushåldz Underwijsning För 40 Åhr sedan Förswänskat Och i många Rum uthaf andra authoribus amplificerat och förbättrat af Isaaco Erici, Pastore Stenbyense i Östergötland*. Stockholm, 1683.

Flintberg, Jacob Albrecht. *Apothekares Badares och Chirurgers Förmoner och Skyldigheter i Stöd av Författningar*. Stockholm, 1786.

Forsius, Sigfrid Aronius. *Almanah eller Dagharäkning* [*1608*]. Stockholm, [1607].

Forsius, Sigfrid Aronius. *Almanah eller Dagharäkning medh thes wahl, wedherlek, sampt flere infälle af then Astronomiska konst och Naturlighe orsakers grunde til thet åhr Christi MDCIX* [*1609*]. Stockholm, [1608].

Fuhrman, Stephanus. *Almanach, På thet Åhret effter wårs Herres Jesu Christi Nåde rijke Födelse 1675*. Stockholm, [1674].

Fuhrman, Stephanus. *Almanach, På thet tänckwördige Skått-Åhret Effter wårs Herres och Frelsares Jesu Christi hugnelige och frögdefulla Födelse 1676*. Stockholm, [1675].

Gyllenius, Petrus Magnus. *Diarium Gylleanium eller Petrus Magnui Gyllenii dagbok 1622–1667*. Edited by Reinh. Hausen. Helsinki: J. Simelii arfvingars tryckeri, 1882.

Haartman, Johan. *Tydelig underrättelse, om de mäst gångbara sjukdomars kännande och motande*. Åbo, 1765.

Harpesträng, Henrik. 'Här byrias läkedombir aff mästher henrik harposträng.' In *Läke- och örteböcker från Sveriges medeltid, första häftet*, edited by G. E. Klemming. Samlingar utg. Af Svenska Fornskrift-Sällskapet, 26. Stockholm: Kongl. Boktryckeriet, 1883.

[Herlicius, David. *Almanac for 1622*. Stockholm, 1621].

Herlicius, David. *Almanach Til thet Ååret Jesu Christi 1632*. Stockholm, [1631].

Herlicius, David. *Calendarium eller Almanach och lille Prognosticon På thet Ååret Jesu Christi Bördh M.DC.XXIII*. Stockholm, [1622].

Kexlerus, Simon. *Almanach Til det ååret effter wår Herres och Frelsares Jesu Christi nåderijka födelses tijd, M.DC. XXXII*. Stockholm, [1631].

Lemnius, Vilhelmus. *Emoot pestilentzie huru hwar och een menniskia sigh hålla skal, bådhe gamble och vnge, rijke och fattige, til itt tiensteligit rådh och hielp, scriffuit genom Guilielmum Lemnium medicinæ doctorem*. Stockholm, 1572.

Lindh, Carl. *Huusz-apoteek och läkie-book*. Visingsborg, 1675.

Magnus, Olaus. *Historia om de nordiska folken*. Uppsala: Michaelisgillet, 1909.

Olai, Benedictus. *Een Nyttigh Läkere Book ther uthinnen man finner rådh, hielp och Läkedom til allehanda menniskiornes siwkdomar bådhe inwertes och uthwertes.* Stockholm, 1578.

Ödmann, Samuel. *Hågkomster från Hembygden och skolan m.m.* Stockholm: A. B. Fahlkrantz Boktryckeri, 1924.

Paulinus Gothus, Laurentius. *Loimoscopia, eller pestilentz speghel. Thet är: Andeligh och naturligh underwiisning, om pestilentzies beskriffwelse, orsaker, praeserwatiiff, läkedomar och befriielser.* Strängnäs, 1623.

Petri, Laurentius. *Then swenska kyrkeordningen.* Stockholm, 1571.

Quensel, Conrad. *Almanach På Åhret efter Jesu Christi Nåderijka Födelse 1724.* Stockholm, 1723.

Rolandsson Martin, Anton. 'Physiologiska Rön och Anmärkningar, om de i Finland hos Almogen brukeliga Badstugors nytta och skada.' *Svenska Vetensk. Acad. Handl.* (1765): 69–77.

Schomerus, Petrus Andreas. *Almanach Til det ååret efter wår Herres och Frelsares Jesu Christi nåderijka födelses tijd, M.DC. XXXII.* Stockholm, [1631].

Spole, Anders. *Almanach På thet Åhret effter Jesu Christi nåderijka födelse til Werlden 1692.* Gothenburg, 1691.

Stenberg, Pehr. *Pehr Stenbergs levernesbeskrivning*, edited by Fredrik Elgh, Göran Stenberg, and Ola Wennstedt, 4 vols. Umeå: Forskningsarkivet vid Umeå universitet, 2014.

Stockholms stads ordinantier påbud och publicationer, edited by Magnus Lagerström, vol. 1. Stockholm, 1731.

Wolff, Valentin. *Späda barns nödiga ans och skötsel, alla christeliga föräldrar åliggande.* Stockholm, 1755.

Digitised works

Gender and Work (*GaW*), Uppsala University, https://gaw.hist.uu.se/. Accessed 20 September 2022.
Case no. 9290.
Case no. 5387.

Literature

Annola, Johanna, Annelie Drakman, and Marie Ulväng, eds. *Med tvål, vatten och flit: Hälsofrämjande renlighet som ideal och praktik ca 1870–1930.* Lund: Nordic Academic Press, 2021.

Bell, Sarah, Ronan Foley, Frank Houghton, Avril Maddrell, and Allison M. Williams. 'From Therapeutic Landscapes to Healthy Spaces, Places and Practices: A Scoping Review.' *Social Science and Medicine* 196 (2018): 123–130.

Bourke, Joanna. 'Pain: Metaphor, Body, and Culture in Anglo-American Societies between the Eighteenth and Twentieth Centuries.' *Rethinking History* 18, no. 4 (2014): 475–498.

Bourke, Joanna. *The Story of Pain: From Prayer to Painkillers*. Oxford: Oxford University Press, 2014.

Carlsson, Lizzie. 'Om badstugor och bad i äldre tid.' *RIG – Kulturhistorisk tidskrift* 30, no. 3 (1947): 113–141.

Collins, Julie. *The Architecture and Landscape of Health: A Historical Perspective on Therapeutic Places, 1790–1940*. London: Routledge, 2020.

Curman, Carl. *Om bad: Om Romerska bad och finska badstugor*. Stockholm: P. A. Norstedt & söner, 1871.

Drakman, Annelie. *När kroppen slöt sig och blev fast: Varför åderlåtning, miasmateori och klimatmedicin övergavs vid 1800-talets mitt*. Uppsala: Acta Universitatis Upsaliensis, 2018.

Duden, Barbara. *The Woman beneath the Skin: A Doctor's Patients in Eighteenth-Century Germany*. Cambridge, MA: Harvard University Press, 1991.

Dvorjetski, Estee. *Leisure, Pleasure and Healing: Spa Culture and Medicine in Ancient Eastern Mediterranean*. Amsterdam: Brill, 2007.

Fors, Hjalmar. 'Medicine and the Making of a City: Spaces of Pharmacy and Scholarly Medicine in Seventeenth-Century Sweden.' *Isis* 107, no. 3 (2016): 473–494.

Forss, Charlotta. *The Old, the New and the Unknown: The Continents and the Making of Geographical Knowledge in Seventeenth-Century Sweden*. Turku: Illoinen Tiede, 2018.

Forss, Charlotta. 'Some Like It Hot: Sex and the Sauna in Early Modern Sweden.' *NOTCHES: – (re)marks on the history of sexuality* (March 2019). http://notchesblog.com/2019/03/19/some-like-it-hot-sex-and-the-sauna-in-early-modern-sweden/. Accessed 10 September 2022.

Gesler, Wilbert M. 'Therapeutic Landscapes: Medical Issues in Light of the New Cultural Geography.' *Social Science and Medicine* 32, no. 7 (1992): 735–756.

Healy, Margaret. 'Why Me? Why Now? How?: The Body in Health and Disease.' In *A Cultural History of the Human Body in the Renaissance*, edited by Linda Kaloff and William Bynum, 37–54. London: Bloomsbury Academic, 2010.

Herbert, Amanda E. 'Gender and the Spa: Space, Sociability and Self at British Health Spas, 1640–1714.' *Journal of Social History* 43 (2009): 361–383.

Hjelt, Otto E. A. *Svenska och finska medicinalverkets historia 1663–1812*, 2 vols. Helsinki: Helsingfors centraltryckeri, 1891.

Jensen, Phebe. *Astrology, Almanacs, and the Early Modern English Calendar*. New York: Routledge, 2020.

Kjellgren, Martin. *Taming the Prophets: Astrology, Orthodoxy and the Word of God in Early Modern Sweden*. Lund, Sekel Bokförlag, 2011.

Klemming, G. E., and E. Eneström. *Svenska almanachor, kalendrar och kalendariska skrifter intill 1749*. Stockholm: P. A. Norstedt & Söner, 1878.

Lindberg, Bo S. *Kirurgernas historia: Om badare, barberare och fältskärer*. Uppsala: Uppsala University, 2017.

Lindemann, Mary. *Medicine and Society in Early Modern Europe*. Cambridge: Cambridge University Press, 2010.

Miglietti, Sara. 'Climate Theory: An "Invented Tradition"?' In *Spreading Knowledge in a Changing World*, edited by Charles Burnett and Pedro Mantas-España, 205–224. Córdoba: Córdoba University Press, 2019.

Miller, Genevieve. '"Airs, Waters, and Places" in History.' *Journal of the History of Medicine and Allied Sciences* 17, no. 1 (1962): 129–140.

Moreau, Elisabeth. 'Complexion, Temperament and Four Humor Theory in the Renaissance.' In *Encyclopedia of Renaissance Philosophy*, edited by Marco Sgarbi. Cham, Switzerland: Springer, 2020. https://doi.org/10.1007/978-3-319-02848-4.

Newton, Hannah. 'Inside the Sickchamber in Early Modern England: The Experience of Illness through Six Objects.' *English Historical Review* 136, no. 580 (2021): 530–567.

Nordenmark, N. V. E. *Naturvetenskapernas historia i Sverige intill år 1800, del 2: Astronomiens historia i Sverige till år I800*. Lychnosbiblioteket 17.2. Uppsala: Almqvist & Wiksell, 1959.

Nordström, Ulrica. *Nordiska bad: I sjö, bassäng och källa*. Stockholm: Natur & Kultur, 2019.

North, Susan. *Sweet and Clean? Bodies and Clothes in Early Modern England*. Oxford: Oxford University Press, 2020.

Ordahl Kupperman, Karen. 'The Puzzle of the American Climate in the Early Modern Period.' *The American Historical Review* 87, no. 5 (1982): 1262–1289.

Roper, Lyndal. 'Martin Luther's Body: '"The Stout Doctor" and His Biographers.' *The American Historical Review* 115, no. 2 (2010): 351–384.

Rublack, Ulinka. 'Fluxes: The Early Modern Body and the Emotions.' *History Workshop Journal* 53 (2002): 1–16.

Runefelt, Leif. *Hushållningens dygder: Affektlära, hushållningslära och ekonomiskt tänkande under svensk stormaktstid*. Stockholm: Almqvist & Wiksell International, 2002.

Runesson, Anton. 'Blod, kött och tårar. Kroppslig erfarenhet i Sverige, ca 1600–1750.' PhD diss., Stockholms universitet, 2021.

Semerdjian, Elyse. 'Naked Anxiety: Bathhouses, Nudity, and the "Dhimmī" Woman in 18th-century Aleppo.' *International Journal of Middle East Studies* 45, no. 4 (2013): 651–676.

Skeri, Karin. *Renlighet och bekvämlighet på Skokloster*. Bålsta: Skoklosters slott, 1992.

Smith, Virginia. *Clean: A History of Personal Hygiene and Purity*. Oxford: Oxford University Press, 2007.

Stolberg, Michael. 'Sweat. Learned Concepts and Popular Perceptions 1500–1800.' In *Blood, Sweat and Tears: The Changing Concepts of Physiology from Antiquity into Early Modern Europe*, edited by Manfred Horstmanshoff, Helen King, and Claus Zittel, 503–522. Leiden: Brill, 2012.

Strandberg, Hindrik. *Koppning i Finland fram till mitten av 1900-talet.* Helsinki: University of Helsinki, 2012.

Swedish Academy Dictionary (*SAOB*). Online: https://www.saob.se/in-english/.

Talve, Illmar. 'Bastu och badstugor.' *Fataburen* (1970): 55–68.

Talve, Illmar. *Bastu och torkhus i Nordeuropa.* Stockholm: Nordiska Museets Handlingar 53, 1960.

Toivo, Raisa Maria. 'Discerning Voices and Values in the Finnish Witch Trials Records.' *Studia Neophilologica* 84, no. 1 (2012): 143–155.

Troels-Lund, Troels Frederik. *Dagligt liv i Norden i det sekstende aarhundrede.* Köpenhamn, 1914.

Van Bavel, Bas, 'The Economic Origins of Cleanliness in the Dutch Golden Age.' *Past & Present* 205 (2009): 41–69.

Van Gent, Jaqueline. *Magic, Body and Self in Eighteenth-Century Sweden.* Leiden: Brill, 2009.

Vigarello, Georges. *Concepts of Cleanliness: Changing Attitudes in France Since the Middle Ages.* New York: Cambridge University Press, 1988.

Wallis, Faith. 'Medicine in Medieval Calendar Manuscripts.' In *Manuscript Sources of Medieval Medicine: A Book of Essays,* edited by Margaret R. Schleissner, 105–143. London and New York: Routledge, 2013.

Wear, Andrew. 'Place, Health, and Disease: The Airs, Waters, Places Tradition in Early Modern England and North America.' *Journal of Medieval and Early Modern Studies* 38, no. 3 (2008): 443–465.

Wiell, Karolina. *Bad mot Lort och Sjukdom: Den privathygieniska utvecklingen i Sverige 1880–1949*. Uppsala: Uppsala University, 2018.

About te Author

Charlotta Forss is an Associate Senior Lecturer, Department of Historical and Contemporary Studies, Södertörn University. Her current research examines how notions of health and morality were renegotiated in the early modern bathhouse culture of Sweden and Finland. Her upcoming book, *Mapping the idea of North* (Oxford: Bodleian Publishing, 2025) explores the connection between conceptions of climate and people on maps.

4. 'Somewhat Heated, Quick and Lively': Humoral Explanations of the Learning Difficulties of Charles XI of Sweden (1655–1697)

Andreas Hellerstedt

Abstract
This chapter explores the education of King Charles XI. The king struggled when learning to read and his teacher struggled to understand and alleviate his pupil's difficulties. The teacher claimed that the king's difficulties were a result of a heroic talent, characteristic of monarchs. Deterministic views of individual talent could serve to reinforce the hierarchical relations of seventeenth-century estate society, but it could also benefit a few talented men from the lower orders. Even in a king, the expectation of innate talent had a meritocratic side, incompatible with hereditary monarchy. The young king was expected to have an exceptional talent, but when this turned out to be unsuitable for academic study, political ideology and pedagogical theory conflicted, while also being unhelpful to the royal pupil.

Keywords: learning difficulties, ingenium, talent, Charles XI of Sweden, Emund Gripenhielm

Introduction

In this chapter, I will explore medical ideas in the context of royal instruction in Sweden during the seventeenth century. In particular, I will look at the young Charles XI, well known as the king who introduced absolutism in Sweden during the latter part of his reign, which lasted for thirty-seven years (1660–1697). Long before that, while the country was still ruled by a regency government during his minority, the boy king Charles struggled

Eyice, M. and C. Forss (eds.), *Health and Society in Early Modern Sweden*.
Taylor & Francis Group 2024
DOI 10.5117/9789463724296_CH04

with learning how to read. This chapter will examine how the king's teacher tried to explain Charles's difficulties by using the medical and pedagogical concepts of the period. Emund Figrelius Gripenhielm (1622–1675) had been chosen as Charles's tutor by the king's father, who had already employed Figrelius for other important tasks.[1] Figrelius was appointed by Charles X on his deathbed, and was ennobled under the name Gripenhielm when he became the young king's teacher. Prior to that, Figrelius had been a university professor, but also an active diplomat and secretary in the royal chancery. Already as a student at Uppsala, Figrelius had worked as a tutor to a young aristocrat. Together with his student, he had undertaken a five-year grand tour of Europe.[2] This provided ample experience as a private teacher.

Learning difficulties is a particularly interesting topic in terms of seventeenth century medical theory. It has been argued that minor variations of temperament were considered normal, and not within the purview of a physicians' profession. To put it more bluntly, there was no cure for stupidity or dull wits, and therefore no reason to administer treatment. Medical doctors generally steered well clear of cases of intellectual disability in the medieval and early modern periods because they were regarded as incurable and the condition as innate and natural.[3] Furthermore, educators largely did the same in a period when only a limited segment of society was required to obtain an education.[4] But a royal student could not be dismissed as unfit for academic study, at least not lightly. And although there were no doctors involved, a 'diagnosis' of sorts was made for Charles XI. In that sense, his case resembles others discussed in this volume (e.g., Anton Runesson's and Charlotta Forss's chapters) in that the medical explanations are closely related to the functions the person was expected to perform. The king was a professional ruler, and as such his difficulties caused concern because they impaired his ability to work.

The conceptual history of learning difficulties

It is clear that the education of the young king became a battleground where political, pedagogical, and even theological issues came to a head. The medical theories that were used to explain the king's shortcomings were strongly affected by these intersecting ideological interests. That fact also

1 Dahlgren, 'Emund Gripenhielm'; MS KB A987a, 1r.
2 Dahlgren, 'Emund Gripenhielm.'
3 Metzler, *Fools and Idiots*, 53–58.
4 Metzler, '"Will-Nots" and "Cannots,"' 55.

illustrates just how flexible and situation-dependent humoral medicine could be. Thus, the context in which humoral theory was employed must always be taken into account if we are to understand it and its historical significance. Arguably, the case of Charles XI illustrates that humoral discourse was much more than a medical theory. It permeated both politics and education in the seventeenth century, as is equally clear from several of the other chapters in this volume. But conversely, it also illustrates how ideas about absolute kingship informed humoral theory in ways that have not always been given due consideration in the history of medicine.

The question of terms and concepts is always a difficult one when it comes to intellectual history in general and the history of medicine in particular. Present-day scholars generally agree that historical concepts, such as the medical diagnoses and pedagogical terminology discussed here, are socially constructed. This does not rule out the existence of transhistorical 'pathologies' as the basis for such conceptualisations, although they may be just as difficult to reach as Kant's famous thing-in-itself. More importantly though, claiming that a concept is socially constructed does not necessarily make us any wiser. It is rather in writing the history of the concepts that we begin to understand *how* terms and concepts were so constructed.[5] The case I discuss in this chapter has previously been subjected to a 'retrodiagnosis.' Retrospective diagnoses of historical subjects are generally problematic and controversial. I will not attempt one here, as my aim is to study the concepts themselves as used in a highly interesting historical context.[6] Consequently, I will use the present-day term 'learning difficulties' in a broad and non-technical sense. When describing and analysing the case of the young Charles's education, I will use the term 'learning difficulties' alongside the historical terms present in the source material. Hopefully, this will shed some light on the concepts themselves, as it is only in use that their significance can be successfully unravelled.

Education for a great power

By the middle of the seventeenth century, Sweden had become one of the great powers of Europe. The spectacular victories during the reigns of

5 McDonagh, Goodey, and Stainton, 'Introduction.'

6 Lindemann, *Medicine and Society*, 9. This does not mean that I disagree with the findings of the study by Åberg and Granström. It may well be true that Charles was what we today would have called 'dyslexic'; the evidence certainly seems convincing.

Gustavus Adolphus, Christina, and Charles X bestowed on the northern kingdom territorial gains to the south, west, and east. In 1660, Sweden was at the height of its geopolitical powers and the kingdom reached its greatest territorial extent. At the same time, Sweden rapidly developed into a modern 'military state,' creating an administration and bureaucracy to match and support the power it projected both nationally and internationally. During this time, the country was also characterised by internal struggles between the monarchy and aristocracy for administrative supremacy in government. Thus, while Sweden was at the height of its power, it also experienced periodic problems of government. These problems were particularly acute both during and after the aristocratically dominated governments that ruled during the long minorities of young rulers such as Christina (1632–1644) and Charles XI (1660–1672). In Sweden, as in the rest of early modern Europe, the elites of the seventeenth century saw a young and impressionable king as an opportunity to be seized. Through education, it was hoped, absolutist tendencies could be held in check, or advanced, as the case may have been. Crown princes were, from a very young age, entangled by political factions, just as they had been entangled by religious factions in the preceding century. However, surprisingly often, the efforts by politicians to mould heirs to the throne after their desired ideals simply failed. Famously, the education of James VI of Scotland (as James I of England), produced the opposite of the political views his teachers wished to inculcate, and in turn, James's own efforts to steer his sons Henry and Charles did not prevent either of them from diverging from their father's intent, which they did, in diametrically opposed directions. In France, Louis, le Grand Dauphin, seems to have developed a hatred of learning from the strict discipline he was subjected to by his teachers, Bossuet and the Duke of Montausier.[7]

The new Swedish state, which had only gained independence from Denmark in the early sixteenth century, made significant efforts to become a great power in the cultural sphere to match its military and political achievements. All of the above-mentioned developments melded together in the field of education. After the Lutheran reformation, Swedish schools were almost abandoned, and the sole university at Uppsala lay dormant for several years. However, the government soon perceived a problem and invested heavily in the educational system. Well-functioning schools and universities were both a source of cultural prestige and an important part in the building of the modern state. The expanding administration of the

7 Pollnitz, *Princely Education*, ch. 6 and 7; Meyer, *L'education des princes*, 20, 113, 134–137, 149–152.

Swedish monarchy required large numbers of educated civil servants.[8] All over Europe, early modern society underwent rapid differentiation, and education had to provide differentiated skills and competencies to match this development.[9] Consequently, the seventeenth century saw the establishment of new schools and universities. Gymnasia were founded on the German model, beginning in Västerås (1623). New universities were founded, in Tartu in Swedish Estonia (1632), Åbo in Finland (1640), and Lund in the former Danish province of Scania (1666). Primary education also expanded greatly, with town and village schools and, most importantly, so-called *husförhör*, catechetical examinations conducted by parish priests with their parishioners in their homes. Exact numbers are hard to come by, but there is reason to believe that literacy in Sweden was among the highest in Europe by the end of the seventeenth century, despite the fact that the vast majority of the population lived in poverty.[10]

These social changes also affected the monarchy. Sweden had a tradition of strong personal rule from the time of Gustav I (r. 1523–1560) onwards, and the general trend in Europe was towards a strong monarchy at the head of a centralised state. These developments in political practice and ideology meant that the demands on the personal capabilities of the monarch were heightened. It is quite appropriate to speak of a professionalisation of the monarchy in the seventeenth century.[11] In order to engage in a meaningful way with the daily business of government, a king had to have at least some knowledge of a wide range of subjects, such as theology, geography, law, history, languages, science, engineering, and the art of war, as well as other subject areas. The institution of hereditary monarchy (established in Sweden in 1544) provided the immediate context for this new form of education. Because the heir was born into his role, there was great opportunity for teachers to prepare their royal pupils with the necessary skills and knowledge required for a monarch. Consequently, an ambitious royal educational program developed during the late sixteenth century to ensure that the young princes (and princesses) received the best that late Renaissance humanist pedagogues could offer. This programme was further developed

8 On these developments, see (for instance) Sjöstrand, *Pedagogikens historia*, 105–325; Sellberg, *Kyrkan och den tidigmoderna staten*, 110–112, 370–371, 382–387, 389–390; Lindroth, *Svensk lärdomshistoria*, 2:37, 41–47.

9 This theme is prominent in Bantock, *Studies in the History*.

10 Admittedly, as a consequence of the unique system of catechetical examinations, Sweden is also one of the few countries for which reliable evidence exists; see, e.g., Houston, 'Literacy and Society.'

11 Meyer, *L'education des princes*, 121–127.

in the seventeenth century, but many of its principles were consistent over a long period of time.

Gustav I had received only a rudimentary education, limited to the Swedish and German languages, religion, and some practical skills such as arithmetic. His sons, on the other hand, were given the benefits of a broad educational programme, including classical languages, natural science, and theology. They were taught by distinguished royal tutors specifically hired for this prestigious task. In the beginning of the seventeenth century, the humanist influenced program became even more ambitious, as is evidenced in the educations of Gustavus Adolphus, Christina, and Charles X. By this time, the programme included not only classical and modern languages, but also history, geography, jurisprudence, politics, rhetoric, moral philosophy, theology, and natural science. Consequently, when Charles X unexpectedly died at age thirty-seven in 1660, the education of the five-year-old heir to the throne (Charles XI) was a grave matter of state which placed very high expectations both on the royal pupil and on his tutors.

As mentioned above, educational plans drawn up for young princes provide valuable insights into royal instruction in Sweden in the early modern period. Such plans exist from the time of the sons of Gustav I and onwards, and have attracted some scholarly attention. The Swedish plans are similar to those found in the Protestant states of northern Germany, Denmark and Britain.[12] Contemporary dissertations on education from Swedish universities is another relevant type of source material, but these have received almost no attention in previous research. Not only were pedagogical issues discussed in these dissertations; the royal tutors – who often had an academic background – also wrote such works themselves. Furthermore, one of the most prominent of the issues they discussed is that of the individual talent of pupils. Why were different people intellectually disposed to different branches of study, how were talents to be discovered and how should a teacher approach students with different talents (*ingenia*, or wits, as they were called in English at the time) were some of the questions that were discussed. It seems that these discussions are connected to what Goodey has described as the increased importance of intelligence: the slow emergence of a meritocracy of abstract thought, which gradually replaced

12 Some important studies are Annell, *Erik XIV:s etiska föreställningar*; Åslund, *Att fostra en kung*; Skuncke, *Gustaf III: det offentliga barnet*. Internationally, see Hoffman, *Raised to Rule*; Müsegades, *Fürstliche Erziehung*; Olden-Jørgensen, '"Herremand I kongeklaeder"'; and Pollnitz, *Princely Education*. Meyer, *L'education des princes*, provides an European overview and some comparisons.

hierarchies of divine grace and social standing during the course of the seventeenth century.[13]

These issues were indeed widely discussed in the seventeenth century. In Sweden, the changes in society and education meant that people from the lower rungs of society could rise through the bureaucracy on the strength of their education, their skills and, not least, their *talent*. The moral philosophical issue of the true nature of nobility and its relation to virtue is one well-known expression of this matter. But there was also a more specifically pedagogical discussion around this phenomenon. This is what was called the problem of *delectus ingeniorum*, the selection of talents. The early modern state increasingly viewed the population as a form of resource. Consequently, the intellectual talents of subjects were also such resources, and the state needed to discover the best of them to use them to maximum advantage. The most extreme proponent of this view was the sixteenth-century Spanish medical doctor Juan Huarte, who argued that individual talent was more or less wholly determined by the physical temperament of the body, and that the state should therefore direct pupils to the appropriate studies and occupations based on medico-pedagogical examinations. Huarte was well known and his ideas influential across Europe, in both Catholic and Protestant countries. Compared to earlier Renaissance educators, such as Erasmus, Huarte represents a distinctly pessimistic and a more deterministic strand of thought.[14]

The plan

A plan was drawn up for the education of young king Charles, one which was just as ambitious as would be expected at that time. In fact, compared to the French education of princes, the Swedish (and German) plans seem to place more emphasis on academic study, especially on languages.[15] The plan for Charles was in many respects a carbon copy of the plan for Christina's studies.[16] It is clear from all these documents that academic studies had become indispensable for a modern monarch, and Charles

13 Goodey, *A History of Intelligence*, in particular ch. 3–7. Goodey also gives a good overview of the conceptual history of ingenium/wit.

14 Huarte's work was translated into Latin as *Scrutinium Ingeniorum*; see also Goodey, *A History of Intelligence*, 73; Kühlmann, *Gelehrtenrepublik und Fürstenstaat*, 340–341; Bantock, *Studies in the History*, 26.

15 Cfr Meyer, *L'education des princes*, 128–132.

16 Åslund, *Att fostra en kung*, 180–183.

XI was expected to master a great number of academic disciplines, but particularly the subjects of religion, ethics, politics, history, geography, languages, and natural sciences.

The education plan, termed an 'Instruction,' provides some background to the educational context Gripenhielm and the young king found themselves in. It was written in 1663, when Charles was eight years old, and his education had already begun. It warns of the risks of young princes being led astray by flatterers who tell them they are subjected to no one and may do whatever they like.[17] The teacher should therefore admonish his student that he will answer to God for his actions. The document itself begins by stressing that the welfare of the whole kingdom depends on the king's education.[18] The instruction is also permeated by the prominent Protestant idea that a king's ability to rule is granted him by the grace of God. Consequently, the king's education should first and foremost focus on religion, and his 'prudence' in the art of government should be informed by his Christian ethics and virtuous personal conduct.[19]

Worldy 'prudence in the business of government' is described thereafter and of primary importance here is languages and rhetoric. The king is expected to acquire proficiency in Swedish and German (which he already knows). He should also have some knowledge of Finnish, which is the language of many of his subjects. Furthermore, French is now so common that it is 'almost' necessary, but Slavic languages are more of an 'ornament' than of any real use. Latin arose out of a noble nation, it has produced an eminent literature, and it is in wide use in Europe, and therefore the king must acquire the 'full knowledge and use' of that language. The instruction also provides some pedagogical pointers. For example, reading the classical authors should be experienced as 'play and enjoyment,' and by reading passages in Swedish beforehand, the teacher can excite 'great lust and appetite' for reading the originals.[20] In general, Gripenhielm should adapt his teaching to the king's status, his age, and the subject at hand. It is important that he strikes a good balance between extremes. On the one hand, he must not tire the young king with excessive study, but on the other, he must not cause him to give up on his studies through 'some neglect and indulgence.' Erasmus's *Institutio Principis Christiani* is pointed to as a pedagogical guide (whereas more modern writers provide the specific content, e.g., on the art of government).[21]

17 MS A987a, 1v.
18 MS A987a, 1v, 1r.
19 MS A987a, 2v–7v, 10v.
20 MS A987a, 7v–9v.
21 MS A987a, 16r–18v.

'His Royal Majesty's reading is somewhat late'

As it happened, the young king struggled tremendously. He was distracted and easily lost interest, while he was more at ease when riding and hunting. Perhaps some of these problems influenced the instruction itself. With time, the king seems to have applied himself more to his academic studies, but matters still did not improve much. Something was clearly amiss with the king's studies. In particular, it had to do with his reading. As the plan for his language studies was very ambitious, this was problematic indeed. The intention was for the king to learn three or more foreign languages, including a strong emphasis on the reading and writing of classical Latin. In fact, the king struggled with reading and writing his native Swedish and German. To complicate matters further, the education of Charles XI was a highly charged political issue, even at his birth. It became even more so when his learning difficulties became known to a wider group.

Not surprisingly, the king's education has been studied by historians for a very long time.[22] One of the claims made very early on (based on rumours that circulated in the seventeenth century) was that the teachers consciously neglected the king's education to ensure that the aristocrats around the king would be able to continue to control him.[23] The king's governor, the overall head of the king's upbringing, the courtier Christer Horn, was certainly not very competent. He was pressured by the Diet to resign, although he never did. However, the king's preceptor (teacher) Emund Gripenhielm was most likely neither a bad teacher, nor was he an instrument of the aristocratic party. As stated earlier, he was both an experienced diplomat and a prominent humanist scholar. After he had begun his personal rule, Charles continued to show Gripenhielm great favour. The king does not seem to have blamed his teacher for his academic failings. On the contrary, Gripenhielm was part of a group of important advisors who contributed to the development of absolutism in the latter part of Charles' reign.[24]

In 1960, historian Alf Åberg and physician K. O. Granström together presented the theory that Charles XI had been dyslexic.[25] They based this on surviving notes written in the king's hand, and on the reports authored by the teacher Gripenhielm, which noted that the king apparently succeeded

22 Schröder/Robson, *Observationes*; Geijer, *Bidrag till historien*, and more recently, Losman, 'Tre karlars studier.'

23 Geijer, *Bidrag till historien*, 6–7.

24 E.g., Rystad, *Karl XI*; Upton, *Charles XI*, 18–19.

25 Åberg and Granström, 'Kunglig ordblindhet.'

well in retelling what he heard and was able to learn many things by heart, but struggled with reading. Furthermore, the king's spelling, even as an adult, was characterised by letters transposed seemingly at random. However, concepts such as 'dyslexia,' 'word-blindness,' and 'specific learning disability' were created in the late nineteenth and early twentieth centuries. These were not terms used by Gripenhielm when trying to understand the king's learning difficulties.

For Gripenhielm, the problem was a question of talent or wit (*ingenium*). In the seventeenth century, such an individual talent was generally thought of as stemming from a person's temperament. This of course is a reference to the mixture of the four fluids of Galenic medical theory. A person's *ingenium* was based on the same 'unified condition' of body and mind which was considered the basis for mental health in general.[26] A fiery temperament would equal a sharp and fast-moving intellect; a wet and cold temperament would make one slow and 'dull-witted.'[27] This medical theory is significant for the education of Charles XI as well. Gripenhielm, and perhaps also others around him, interpreted the king's learning difficulties as a result of his unique individual temperament. This is something that has been largely overlooked in previous research. Moreover, it was not just that Gripenhielm considered the king to have a certain temperament which could explain his difficulties. Gripenhielm also attached highly interesting *political* ideas to this particular type of talent.

Gripenhielm had made some remarks on the nature of different talents both in the works from his period as a professor at Uppsala and during his time as royal preceptor. First, I will look at what he said when questioned by the Privy Council and Diet about his student's progress.

In June 1663, Gripenhielm claims that he had observed 'a particular *indoles* in his Majesty,' which would develop well if only the king had some good co-students to accompany him when studying.[28] *Indoles* is one of the

26 As discussed in Riikka Miettinen's chapter in this volume.

27 Edlund, 'Temperamentsläran som begåvningsteori.'

28 The quote reads as follows in the original: 'Orsaken dertill, att det går något sent med H. K. M:ts läsande [...] utan det synes bestå uti H. K. M:ts egen gemöts disposition, som är af naturen något hetsigt, prompt och lefvandes, och esomoftast blandar tankarne tillhopa med hvarandra, och praecipiterar dem hvar öfver annan, hvarigenom sker något hinder uti det som för händer hafves, ehuru stor flit man ock gör sådant både med lindrigare och allvarsamme remonstrationer att betaga. Till hvilket allt är ett infallibelt märke, att H. M:t efter iläsandet beygnner ordet af den siste bokstafven och stundom af den som midt i ordet står; hvarföre mest man förhoppas af tiden, att hon lärer afgöra derutinnan en god verkning: Nam in tali Casu, quantacunque Cura vel Industria Informatoris, ministra solum est Natura[e], non Domina.' Geijer, *Bidrag till historien*, 11. All translations in this chapter are my own.

terms used in the pedagogical literature of the time to describe an innate, natural-born ability, character or constitution. Indeed, the word *indoles* appears on the title page of Gripenhielm's own 1654 dissertation, in which he discusses exactly the question of different types of talent (a point to which I will return shortly). From the start, Gripenhielm was convinced (or tried to convince himself and others) that the king's natural abilities were good, or even excellent.

A couple of years later, in 1665, when Charles was ten, Gripenhielm was asked to explain why the boy-king had had such difficulties learning to read. He says:

> The cause that His Royal Majesty's reading is somewhat late [...] seems to be H. R. M's own disposition of mind [*gemöt*], which is by nature somewhat heated, quick and lively, and he often mixes thoughts with one another, and anticipates them over each other, whereby there is some hindrance in the task that he has at hand, no matter how much diligence is used in both mild and serious remonstrations to remove this. All of which is an infallible mark, that H. M. after reading, begins the word with the last letter and sometimes with the middle; upon which one hopes that time will have a good effect: for in such a case, no matter how much industry and care is heeded by the teacher, he is still only the servant of nature, not its master.[29]

In other words, the king's intellect, which is no doubt very sharp, is just a little too fast in its movement. Already in the Hippocratic texts, sound reason was described as a proper balance between fire and water, where too much fire would result in thinking too quickly, and too much water would cause slow thinking. In the early modern period, the power of reason was increasingly described as being the same as quick-thinking, and labelled 'ingenium,' that is, the earlier ideal of balance shifted towards the extreme of fiery quickness.[30] The same condition which in normal cases of the early modern period would cause superior intelligence has in this particular case caused problems with reading. Rather than ascribing the problem to lack of talent, the teacher here takes it to be the opposite instead. By nature, the king is highly gifted, and this is precisely what is causing him problems.

29 Gripenhielm's response to the Privy Council, 10 March 1665, quoted in Geijer, *Bidrag till historien*, 21.
30 Goodey, *A History of Intelligence*, 54.

The king's education did not progress very far, and the ambitiously laid plans were never fulfilled. By the time he was twelve, the king read Comenius's *Orbis Sensualium Pictus*, the famous picture book meant as a first reader. At fourteen and fifteen, he was reported to be able to read chapters from Cornelius Nepos, one of the first Latin authors beginners would read. By that time, he began to attend Privy Council sessions and soon thereafter his studies ceased. In other words, while the diagnosis was reasonable enough in terms of the theories of the day, the king's difficulty with learning how to read was never overcome. There was a sort of 'diagnosis,' but there was no cure. Gripenhielm hoped that time might work in their favour. This was a reasonable expectation, as temperaments were generally understood to develop with age. However, such a natural development never took place, and the king's difficulties persisted throughout his life.

Finally, I will now turn to look at what Gripenhielm[31] had to say about individual talents before he became the king's teacher. In my view, this is key to understanding Gripenhielm's 'diagnosis' of his pupil. The most relevant material in this context is a dissertation published in 1654. It is a political discourse on the three main types of *ingenium*. Consequently, it provides a *political* view on the issue of talent, quite different from the opinions expressed by educational writers of the period. The various talents are not divided according to academic or professional potential. This is not the perspective of the selection of talents (*delectus ingeniorum*) as commonly understood. Instead, talents are categorised after their political usefulness. And politics, of course, was conceptualised in Roman terms. For example, is this individual just a potential Gracchus, a Marius, or a Sulla – or is he a future Alexander, a Caesar, or an Augustus?

Gripenhielm argues that there are three main types of talent, each with its particular set of characteristics. First, there is the 'vulgar' sort. Persons with this type of talent never reach anything but the lowest of achievements in life. The prudent ruler must, however, learn to know and understand them, because the common people, acting as a mob, can be dangerous. Second, there are the more elevated spirits, who may become prominent citizens. They display great patriotism and virtue but tend to be content with things as they are. Thus, they are more of a middling rank than kings or princes, but may be useful as servants of a ruler.

Third, there are those whose virtue, fate, and fortunes place them at the summit of society in 'a greatness which is rarely bestowed upon mortal

31 At that time, he was not yet ennobled and therefore still named Figrelius. For the sake of readability, I refer to him as Gripenhielm throughout this chapter.

men.'[32] This third category of particularly excellent individuals are known as 'heroes.' They have received the divine gift of a fiery temperament which gives them an exceptional power and energy and a talent in all aspects of life. It is characteristic for them to have not just one or two particular gifts, but many. They exceed others in both military matters and civilian professions. Their heroic character can be observed early in life. It manifests itself physically. Such heroes have fire in their eyes, even sparks around their heads. They act with unexpected speed and no difficulties are insurmountable.

This concept of the superhuman, perfect 'hero' as the ideal for a baroque prince was evident in the time of Charles's son, Charles XII, as well. These kings were portrayed, in pictorial representations and panegyric verse, as Alexanders or Herculeses, as were many monarchs all over Europe in the seventeenth century. However, this ideology took a specific form in Sweden, which was derived from the Strasbourg historian and classicist Johann Heinrich Boeclerus. His influence is clear from direct references and quotations in both Figrelius's dissertation and in similar texts from the days of Charles XII, not least those of his teacher, Andreas Nordenhielm.[33]

It was Boeclerus who forwarded the idea of the political hero, whose penetrating and quick-moving intellect could supposedly distinguish the true causes of things and act in anticipation of his adversaries, making him a perfect ruler. According to Boeclerus, such individuals, modelled on the great rulers of antiquity, were 'by God gifted with an unusual and almost unique and marvellous greatness of talent, and further equipped with a swiftness in the most important arts, and they were destined to carry out important and public duties.'[34]

Boeclerus only spent a couple of turbulent years in Sweden as a professor at Uppsala, but he left a legacy in the form of many important ideas which he passed on to disciples such as Gripenhielm and Nordenhielm. This was an ideology suited to a strong monarchy and fit the requirements of the state when directed towards its subjects and towards its international peers. But the ideologues themselves, and the monarchs they served, became

32 Figrelius/Agraeus, *Discursus Politicus*, 3. The co-author Agraeus was the student who ostensibly defended this dissertation under the supervision of professor Figrelius. In such instances, the professor would often make significant contributions to the text, sometimes being the sole author himself. The exact role of the student and professor is difficult to determine in this case.

33 Figrelius/Agraeus, *Discursus Politicus*, 3–7; Boeclerus's ideas have shaped the entire dissertation, which utilises the same sources (Roman historian Velleius Paterculus, among others). For Charles XII and Nordenhielm, see Hellerstedt, 'The Absolute Hero.'

34 Boeclerus, *Characteres Politici*, r. 7 (the 1672 edition lacks proper pagination).

prisoners of their own ideas. Gripenhielm's theory told him that the king would have a hero's temperament: fiery, quick-thinking, resolute, decisive, like an Alexander cutting the Gordian knot. He could not, or dared not perhaps, imagine that the king's *ingenium* would be a phlegmatic, tardy one. Kings were just not like that. This would otherwise have been the logical conclusion when faced with the difficulties that Charles had. However, as Goodey has pointed out, towards the second half of the seventeenth century, the 'fast model' for intelligence (*ingenium* or wit) was becoming increasingly dominant. And as the purpose of concepts such as *ingenium* was, to a great extent, to draw the line between us and the 'others,' the only option was perhaps to describe Charles XI as a fiery, quick-thinking hero, with appropriately heroic learning difficulties.[35]

Gripenhielm tried to make sense of the king's learning difficulties in terms of his own medicalised view of education, but conversely, his political ideals also shaped his medical concepts. The king must be suffering from an excessively heroic temperament because that was a temperament appropriate for kings. The learning difficulties were, in that sense, described as a 'royal disease' of sorts. The reason why Charles could not easily learn to read was the same reason that enabled Alexander to lead the attack and turn the tide of battle at Issos and the same reason which caused Caesar to cross the Rubicon and secure power over the Roman Empire. Unfortunately, but unsurprisingly, this 'diagnosis' did not help the prince in his studies. It may, however, very well have deflected responsibility away from the teacher while serving to uphold the majestic image of absolute kingship. The young king was indeed described as being fragile and sickly as a boy, and his mother has been blamed for being over-protective to the extent that it affected his studies.[36] However, the fiery temperament described by Gripenhielm does not appear to be connected to the king's ill health, at least not explicitly. Neither is anything mentioned in terms of dietary recommendations or any other interventions which could potentially have cured the condition. It seems likely, as was stated in the introduction to this chapter, that the king's temperament was taken to be a natural one, in the more deterministic sense of, for instance, Huarte. His temperament might develop to some extent during the course of life, but it was, for all practical purposes, fixed.

It is thus doubtful that the king's difficulties were seen as a form of ill health. They were indeed 'diagnosed' in a certain sense, as we have seen from the discussion above. However, there is nothing to indicate that this

35 Goodey, *A History of Intelligence*, 49–59, 69–75.

36 Rystad, *Karl XI*, 23.

was a medical diagnosis in the stricter sense of the term. Nor was it made by a trained physician. Gripenhielm does not seem to connect the king's reading difficulties to his health. Instead, the temperament causing the young king's disability is a hero's temperament, not that of a fragile youth.

Yet the importance of humoral medicine is readily apparent in the case of the king's aptitude for reading. Rather than being a question of health, it points instead to the broader importance of medical theories in seventeenth century life and ideas, as outlined in the introduction to this volume. The four humours shaped conceptions not only of health or disease, but of other, equally fundamental notions of human nature, such as gender, age, individual character, and not least, talent and academic potential. The flexible theory of the humours was also, as is evident in this case, often informed by prevailing relations of power. It was generally shaped to fit the estate system of stratified groups in which it was so influential. However, as always, men of power could themselves be trapped by the expectations to which it subjected them. Having a hero's temperament was, it seems, a mixed blessing, even for a king.

Bibliography

Archival sources

Kungliga biblioteket

Stockholm A987a, 'Instruction, Hwar efter Kongl. Maijttz Praeceptor Emund Gripenhielm, uti Kongl. Maijttz information och lärdom Sig hafwer at regulera och rätta gifwen i Stockholm d. 24 Novembr. Ao: 1663.'

Printed works

Boeclerus, Johann Heinrich. *Characteres Politici in Velleio Paterculo*. Strasbourg, 1672.

Figrelius, Emund/Agraeus, Olaus. *Discursus Politicus De Triplici Ingeniorum Varietate*. Uppsala: diss., Uppsala universitet, 1655.

Huarte, Juan. *Scrutinium Ingeniorum pro ijs, qui Excellere Cupiunt*. Leipzig, 1622.

Literature

Annell, Gunnar. *Erik XIV:s etiska föreställningar och deras inflytande på hans politik*. Uppsala: Uppsala universitet, 1945.

Bantock, Geoffrey Herman. *Studies in the History of Educational Theory*, vol 1. London: Allen & Unwin, 1980.

Dahlgren, Stellan. 'Emund Gripenhielm.' *Svenskt biografiskt lexikon*. https://sok.riksarkivet.se/sbl/artikel/13216. Accessed 24 June 2021.

Edlund, Sven. 'Temperamentsläran som begåvningsteori.' *Vetenskapssocieteten i Lund, årsbok 1947*. Lund: Gleerups, 1947.

Kühlmann, Wilhelm. *Gelehrtenrepublik und Fürstenstaat: Entwicklung und Kritik des deutschen Späthumanismus in der Literatur des Barockzeitalters*. Tübingen: Niemayer, 1982.

Lindemann, Mary. *Medicine and Society in Early Modern Europe*. Cambridge: Cambridge University Press, 2010.

Lindroth, Sten. *Svensk lärdomshistoria*. 4 vols. Stockholm: Norstedts, 1975.

McDonagh, Patrick, C. F. Goodey, and Tim Stainton. 'Introduction: The Emergent Critical History of Intellectual Disability.' In *Intellectual Disability. A Conceptual History 1200–1900*, edited by Patrick McDonagh, C. F. Goodey, and Tim Stainton, 1–25. Manchester: Manchester University Press, 2018.

Metzler, Irina. *Fools and Idiots? Intellectual Disability in the Middle Ages*. Manchester: Manchester University Press, 2016.

Metzler, Irina. '"Will-nots" and "Cannots": Tracing a Trope in Medieval Thought.' In *Intellectual Disability. A Conceptual History 1200–1900*, edited by Patrick McDonagh, C. F. Goodey, and Tim Stainton, 45–63. Manchester: Manchester University Press, 2018.

Meyer, Jean. *L'education des princes du XVe au XIXe siècle*. Paris: Perrin, 2004.

Geijer, Knut. *Bidrag till historien om konung Carl XI:s uppfostran*. Stockholm: diss., Uppsala universitet, 1842.

Goodey, C. F. *A History of Intelligence and 'Intellectual Disability': The Shaping of Psychology in Early Modern Europe*. Farnham: Ashgate, 2011.

Hellerstedt, Andreas. 'The Absolute Hero: Heroic Greatness and Royal Absolutism in Sweden 1685–1715.' In *Shaping Heroic Virtue: Studies in the Art and Politics of Supereminence in Europe and Scandinavia*, edited by Stefano Fogelberg Rota and Andreas Hellerstedt, 153–185. Brill: Leiden, 2015.

Hoffman, Martha K. *Raised to Rule: Educating Royalty at the Court of the Spanish Habsburgs*. Baton Rouge: Louisiana State University Press, 2011.

Houston, Rab. 'Literacy and Society in the West 1500–1850.' *Social History* 8, no. 3 (1983): 269–293.

Losman, Arne. 'Tre karlars studier.' In *Tre karlar: Karl X* Gustav – *Karl XI – Karl XII*, edited by Gudrun Ekstrand, 11–25. Stockholm: Livrustkammaren, 1984.

Müsegades, Benjamin. *Fürstliche Erziehung und Ausbildung im spätmittelalterlichen Reich*. Ostfildern: Thorbecke, 2014.

Olden-Jørgensen, Sebastian. '"Herremand I kongeklaeder" eller "af den gamle skole": Randbemaerkninger til en udgave av Christian IV's brevstile.' *Aigis: Nordisk*

tidsskrift for klassiske studier. Supplementum I (2011): 1–14. https://aigis.igl.ku.dk/aigis/CGT/fsg.ind.html. Accessed 29 September 2022.
Pollnitz, Aysha. *Princely Education in Early Modern Britain.* Cambridge: Cambridge University Press, 2015.
Rystad, Göran. *Karl XI: En biografi.* Lund: Historiska media, 2001.
Schröder, J. H./H. J. Robson. *Observationes circa educationem Caroli XI.* Uppsala: Uppsala universitet, 1836.
Sellberg, Erland. *Kyrkan och den tidigmoderna staten: En konflikt om Aristoteles, utbildning och makt.* Stockholm: Carlssons, 2010.
Sjöstrand, Wilhelm. *Pedagogikens historia,* II. Lund: Gleerups, 1965.
Skuncke, Marie-Christine. *Gustaf III: Det offentliga barnet: En prins retoriska och politiska fostran.* Stockholm: Atlantis, 1993.
Upton, Anthony F. *Charles XI and Swedish Absolutism.* Cambridge: Cambridge University Press, 1998.
Åberg, Alf, and K. O. Granström. 'Kunglig ordblindhet – Karl XI:s läs- och skrivsvårigheter.' *Svenska Läkartidningen* 58, no. 13 (1961): 1–13.
Åslund, Leif. *Att fostra en kung: Om drottning Kristinas utbildning.* Stockholm: Atlantis, 2005.

About the Author

Andreas Hellerstedt is an Associate Professor in the history of ideas and lecturer at Mid Sweden University, Sundsvall. His research focuses on, among other topics, the early modern mirrors for princes and the history of universities.

5. Health in Body and Soul in a Female Birgittine Convent 1516–1522

Gabriela Bjarne Larsson

Abstract

This chapter analyses the perceptions of health of the early modern former spice merchant and Birgittine nun, Katerina Lemmel. At the monastery she entered at age fifty, they combined religious healing methods with humoral pathological methods. Katerina introduced spiced food, salutary drinks, and medication made of spices and a liquid binder. She considered the medicinal effects of using spices in these different ways as equivalent to traditional religious healing methods. They all promoted well-being and contentment, as well as strength. Nevertheless, whether one would remain healthy or recover from an ailment lay in the hands of God. However, an individual should contribute to their own well-being. First and foremost, one should eat the right foods but not abstain from food.

Keywords: spice treatments, healing methods, well-being, Birgittine Rule, bleeding

Introduction

This chapter is an attempt to elucidate how Katerina Lemmel, a newly widowed former spice merchant, who entered a Birgittine nunnary in 1516, perceived sickness and health. I aim to capture her beliefs and experiences, conceptions and comprehensions, of what people in those days called bodily and spiritual health. Furthermore, I examine by what means and methods what we call physical and mental ailments were prevented or combated in the female convent at Maria Mai in Maihingen, Germany. The two key questions I consider are: Were humoral pathological methods combined with religious ones? And how was God's impact on healing perceived?

Eyice, M. and C. Forss (eds.), *Health and Society in Early Modern Sweden.*
Taylor & Francis Group 2024
DOI 10.5117/9789463724296_CH05

I examine the ways in which Katerina contributed to the well-being of her sisters in the female convent, especially how she introduced luxury products such as spices, salutary drinks, and wine as healing products. I also study her view of the impact of faith on sickness, recovery, and death. Katerina's views and beliefs can be identified by reading her letters to her cousin, one of her former associates in the spice trading company that she had been a part of before entering the monastery Maria Mai in Maihingen in 1516. An analysis of her letters gives us, for the first time, an idea of how a nun – specifically a nun from the Swedish Birgittine order – experienced health and healing. She was not herself a healer, but a representative of the enlightened urban population. Throughout her professional life, she lived according to humoral pathological ideas, with the help of the family's own pharmacist. Entering the monastery age fifty, she transferred her experiences and knowledge of health and cures primarily to the female convent at the monastery.

Control or cure the body – or create well-being?

When we enter the second decade of the sixteenth century, medical knowledge is widespread, especially in the European towns, but even in Scandinavian towns and monasteries.[1] An abundance of written medicinal treatises, fasting treatises, vernacular health regimes, herbal books, remedy and recipe books were circulated in handwritten copies, or had even been published.[2] The Birgittine mother house, Vadstena, possessed quite a number of medicinal works. Some of them were copied and sent to other monasteries within the Birgittine order, such as Naantali Monastery, in present-day Finland.[3] During the first two decades of the fifteenth century, Vadstena had a lively exchange with the Birgittine monastery Munkaliv in Bergen, Norway. Munkaliv, in turn, had good contacts with German-speaking areas. Both Vadstena and Munkaliv owned books printed or copied in Nuremberg, the town where Katerina grew up.[4] Reading Katerina's

1 Krötzl, 'Saints,' 262.

2 Uddenberg, 'Boken,' 7–15; Larsson, *Millefolium*, 17–57, Christensen Nugues, 'Skolmedicinen,' 70–72.

3 Vadstena Monastery was located in the middle of the southern part of what was then Sweden. Another Swedish Birgittine monastery in present-day Finland, Naantali, possessed, among other works, a herbal book: *Nadhe(n)dals clost(er)s book*. According to Larsson, this herbal book was written by the Vadstena Monastery and given to Naantali Monastery; see *Millefolium*, 34. See also Niiranen, 'Medical Knowledge,' 42.

4 Carlqvist, 'Abbedissan,' 19–20.

correspondence reveal that she, and her abbess at Maihingen, had many contacts in Bergen.[5] Books were copied and distributed between the Birgittine monasteries, and 'medicinal' works incorporated humoral theory to a greater or lesser degree. Humoral theory explained how diseases arose but also how they could be cured. According to contemporary medical theory, a person developed a disease when the body's humoral temperament was imbalanced.

Food was one of the things that could influence the humours in a negative or in a positive way, and thus food affected health. Spices in particular possessed strong humoral properties.[6] According to humoral theory, spices helped to balance the internal fluids of the body: they were commonly dry, and used in food to counteract negative properties when food was cold or moist. When the humours were in balance, one was healthy.

Spices could also be used as medication because they were considered to prevent or cure disease. A spice was usually dissolved in a liquid, such as vinegar, wine or beer, and served as a beneficial drink. The scent of a spice could also be used by putting it in some kind of vessel or even in amulets.[7] Both in private houses and in churches, a visitor would sense aromatic odours in late medieval Europe, which were used to counteract bad vapours. Moreover, not only taste and odour but also colour were thought to influence the mind and therefore the body, according to medieval thinking.[8] Given the importance of spices and their uses during this period, Katerina Lemmel's use of them at Maihingen is the study's main focus.

It was not only eating bad foods that was damaging to health; being exposed to bad vapours could also cause imbalance in the body. Enlightened people in European towns explained this imbalance by saying that bad vapours had penetrated the pores of the body. Bad smells had similar effects when they penetrated the mind and the rest of the body through the nose.[9] These imbalances were combated with spices – for example, the use of incense. Other external factors that influenced health, which I will partially touch upon, were for example the relationship between sleep–wakefulness, movement (work) – rest, and climate, including air quality, all of which were recognised both in Galenic and Arabic systems of humoral theory.[10]

5 *Pepper for Prayer*, 69, 115, 137, 157.

6 Freedman, *Out of the East*, 52–54; Freedman, 'Health, Wellness,' 47–48 (herbs and spices).

7 Niiranen, 'Mental Disorders.'

8 Freedman, 'Health, Wellness,' 48–49.

9 Niiranen, 'Sexual,' 235; Ritchey and Strocchia, 'Introduction,' 28.

10 Freedman, *Out of the East*, 54; all six external factors are in Ritchey and Strocchia, 'Introduction,' 25; the six with alternative designations are in Boquet and Nagy, *Medieval Sensibilities*, 136–137.

In Sweden, researchers still discuss the extent to which the Swedish monasteries' healthcare efforts reached out to the lay community. Recent research, however, states that the importance of monasteries for medical methods practised outside the convents should be downplayed. Furthermore, in late medieval Sweden, medical instruments (e.g., for bleeding and enemas) were far more common in male monasteries than in female monasteries,[11] and in this chapter, I primarily explore the Maihingen monastery's female convent through Katerina Lemmel. One key question to examine is: Did the nuns in Maihingen use bloodletting and enemas as healing methods?

One factor that especially influenced communities outside the monasteries was the way monks and nuns explained why someone was struck by mental or physical illness. In their explanations, the divine played a crucial role. By praying and having faith, a person could recover as if by a miracle. In humoral theory, on the other hand, the explanations were corporal; the body fluids were out of balance and thus had to be restored. How did Katerina, a former tradeswoman, a burgher, combine these two theories? In what contexts did she explain disease or the properties of spices from a humoral pathological perspective and when did the religious explanations take place?

Another question I pose regarding Katerina's activities has a moral or an ethical edge and perhaps is more relevant for women's monasteries than for men's monasteries. Such a question arises because there seems to have been a stronger ideal among the nuns than among the monks to be ascetic and to abstain from food. *Anorexia mirabilis* (holy anorexia) was much more practised by women than by men, at least during the high Middle Ages. To renounce eating or repress eating was a way of disciplining, manipulating, or controlling the body, so that the mind/soul could be better prepared for meeting with God. Some would say that nuns were renouncing the health of their bodies when fasting, although their goal was to be nearer Christ.[12] If there was still an anorexic ideal revered in Katerina's time and practised by her monastery, how could the import of luxury products, such as spices, sugar, and dried fruit, be defended?

For the last decade or so, researchers have, somewhat to their surprise, observed that at least in the lives of monks in the late Middle Ages, following the Rule of Saint Benedict, it was not in their dietary practice to abstain from

11 Bergqvist, *Läkare och läkande*, 238–244, 260–261, especially 327–331. Bergqvist, *Läkare och läkande*, 299, 302 underlines that bloodletting could be a treatment practised outside real knowledge of humoral pathology in medieval Sweden.

12 Bynum, *Holy Feast*, passim; Vandereycken, *From Fasting Saints*, passim.

food. Lent and other fasting periods only meant eating specific products.[13] Was this perhaps also the case in Katerina's convent? And what does the Rule of Saint Birgitta say about the fasting?

The fact that the latest research has been able to establish that fasting did not necessarily mean refraining from eating, but rather was about eating alternative products, confirms the criticism of the early Protestant reformers. Catholics were criticised by Protestants for being hypocrites when fasting. According to the reformers, true fasting 'required abstinence from all foods and drinks, not just meat.'[14]

The philosopher Henrik Lagerlund states that food ethics in the Middle Ages was very much related to eating or avoiding meat and the moral status of animals, as well as moral principles about eating and drinking too much.[15] Eating too much – gluttony – was a deadly sin and it often led to another sin of the body, namely lust, which has been highlighted by many scholars. In the following study, I am more interested in what Lagerlund calls the second meaning of gluttony, namely to eat too luxuriously, or too exotically, or too expensively.[16] In what ways did Katerina try to avoid the sin of gluttony in this second meaning when she ordered luxury items such as spices for the monastery's two convents?

Medical knowledge and spices as healing or preventing illness

The fact that Katerina had experience as a spice merchant is important. All her life, up until she was fifty years old, she lived in the prosperous town Nuremberg. Her family had for generations owned and managed a trading company that imported spices. When she married, she remained active within her family firm, while her husband had a company that traded in wine and metal. When her husband died, after twenty-nine years of marriage, Katerina chose not to remarry. Instead, in 1516, she entered the Birgittine nunnery in Maihingen.[17] Katerina left all her assets and savings in the hands of her cousin Hans Imhof, who would manage her fortune until he died in 1522. It is the correspondence between the two that is my main source in the following discussion.[18]

13 Musumeci, 'Urban Influence,' 33–34; Threlfall-Holmes, *Munks and Markets*, 220–223.

14 Barnett, 'Reforming Food,' 518.

15 Lagerlund, 'Food Ethics,' 759–772.

16 Lagerlund, 'Food Ethics,' 769.

17 Schier et al., 'Introduction,' 11–12.

18 See *Pepper for Prayer*: the editors have published a lot of research based on this correspondence, for which see the Bibliography at the end of the edition. In the 'Introduction,' uner the

During the first four years at the convent, she wrote almost every month to her cousin Hans, who managed her property and provided her with the goods she asked him to send to the male and female convents at Maihingen monastery. In most cases, she asked him to send specific spices. The letters are a blend of her business transactions with her cousin, descriptions of her spiritual life, and her yearning for family news.

Hans Imhof and his brothers ran the trading company which still traded and imported spices. Moreover, Hans was a prominent 'member of the inner chamber of the Nuremberg city council.'[19] Katerina's family affiliation with the company had given her access to many network contacts and knowledge of marketplaces. In Hans she found a trustworthy and faithful ally who was invaluable in enabling her to procure the goods she wanted for the monastery in Maihingen.[20] The goods were mostly paid with the help of interest income that was derived from her held mortgages and real estate. The fact that she paid for her goods with her own money caused problems for her and the abbess at Maihingen. No nun had the right to own anything. Nevertheless, it was money from Katerina's property (managed by Hans) that paid for the imported goods received at the monastery.[21]

With certainty, Katerina was familiar with the medical uses of spices, whether they were used in food or in medicaments. Both uses were considered to promote health or well-being, even to heal a sick person. We know from her letters that within her family there was an expert on how to use spices for health purposes. Their own 'apothecary,' Uncle Pirckheimer gave family members advice in healing matters and prescribed medicine for ailments.[22] During this period, any spice merchant could be taken for a pharmacist,[23] and Katerina's family had appointed one of their own as a specialist in such matters.

One difficulty that arises when reading Katerina's letters is that she seldom reveals whether the spices ordered should be used for cooking or for medicines, an observation also Threlfall-Holmes made when analysing, in a British context, the accounts for Durham Cathedral Priory.[24] Many of the

heading 'Significance' (18–25), the richness of the letters is presented and research fields are suggested.

19 Schier et al., 'Introduction,' 9.

20 *Pepper for Prayer*, 69, 71.

21 Schier et al., 'Introduction,' 18, touch upon this slightly and say that Katerina was well aware of the prohibition against owning or keeping private wealth and possessions as a Birgittine nun. Some letters in her correspondence deal with these problems.

22 *Pepper for Prayer*, 105, 119.

23 Nam, 'Medieval,' 320.

24 Threlfall-Holmes, *Monks and Markets*, 60.

spices Katerina ordered, such as nutmeg, cloves, ginger, cinnamon, and more, were used both in cooking and for medicinal purposes.[25] Research has shown that some spices and dried fruits were preferably used on special occasions during the liturgical year.[26] Assuming such was the case, I try to determine at what points in time Katerina's request for spices was sent to Hans. If the spices were ordered before a liturgical feast, they would most likely be used in cooking, but could of course be used as a medicinal beverage, too. Did Katerina perceive spices in food differently from spices in medication?

In Nuremberg, a whole range of healing methods were available through many written texts. During this period, it is difficult to separate healing methods from each other in these manuals. The religious and medical were intertwined. It is of little use to call them 'medicinal,' 'occult,' 'religious,' 'medical,' 'experimental,' and so forth. In those days, the use of foods, and especially spices, in healing could be understood as also having 'spiritual' healing powers. However, food, herbals, and spices could also be considered simply as 'natural' matter. Uses and methods were mixed or intertwined and created hybridised forms of care practices.[27]

Another difficulty when interpreting her statements about spices is that Katerina does not explicitly write about whether the use of a certain spice cures the person from illness or only maintains health. I, however, read her comments in light of the assumption that she had humoral pathological knowledge. For Katerina and her contemporaries, this meant that they could not know if a specific person would respond positively to a medication because every person's body and fluid balances appeared differently. In the herbal books of the time, this is shown by the fact that the same ailment could be cured with different spices or herbs. The patient had to experience which combination had the best effect. Since spices possess properties that affect the body's fluids, they promote balance and thus the people of the time believed that the spices could result in being cured. Before reaching a cured state, spices were used to prevent imbalance, and by maintaining a healthy balance once it was achieved.

In addition to manuals on healing, there is evidence of oral transmission. Recent research has been able to state that late medieval town women generally had knowledge of household medicine and practised it on members of the family.[28] Katerina surely acquired this experience during her thirty

25 Freedman, 'Health, Wellness,' 50.

26 Threlfall-Holmes, *Monks and Markets*, 61.

27 Barker and Strocchia, 'Household Medicine,' 140; Dumas, 'L'Ymage,' passim.

28 See articles in: *Gender, Health and Healing, 1250–1550*; also *Infirmity in Antiquity and the Middle Ages*.

years of marriage and brought this knowledge with her when entering the monastery at Maihingen. I agree with Richey and Strocchia that it is likely that Katerina, as a female householder in a city, 'put learned discourse to practical use,'[29] so that when she entered the monastery in Maihingen, she could blend her acquired knowledge and experience with spiritual liturgical practices and the monastery's healing tradition. What came out of Katerina's mixed practice and how she explained the way her treatments enhanced the sister's well-being will be discussed further. But first, an overview of the Birgittine Rule will be presented.

The Birgittine Rule, *Regula Salvatoris*, fasting, and luxurious goods

Katerina had carefully chosen which monastery she wished to enter.[30] It took her three years of preparation and reading before she moved from Nuremberg to Maihingen. It is furthermore most likely that she was acquainted with Saint Birgitta's *Revelationes* before she entered the monastery in Maihingen 1516. The *Revelationes* had been published in Katerina's hometown, Nuremberg, first in Latin in 1500, and later in a Maihingen German translation in 1502. These books reached several destinations in Europe.[31]

In this section I discuss Birgitta's attitude to health through her comments on fasting. *Regula Salvatoris*, the rule that governed everyday life in Birgittine monasteries in medieval Europe includes instructions regarding food, diet, and fasting.[32] 'Copies of the Rule in Latin and German were available at Maria Mai,'[33] and Katerina refers to it a handful of times in the letters. From the letters we can conclude that she really had read and understood the Rule.[34]

In *Regula Salvatoris*, chapter 24, it is stated that you should treat your body as if it were a weak working animal and satisfy its needs, so that you will serve God well. Chapter 9 presents the cycle of fasting periods and feast

29 Ritchey and Strocchia, 'Introduction,' 24.

30 Schier et al., 'Introduction,' 18.

31 Schier et al., 'Introduction,' 12–13.

32 Available at https://litteraturbanken.se/f%C3%B6rfattare/Birgitta/titlar/HimmelskaUppenbarelserIV/sida/7/faksimil in a Swedish translation, otherwise in different medieval copies in Latin.

33 Schier et al., 'Introduction,' 19.

34 *Pepper for Prayer*, letters 26, 29, 32, 35, and 55. In a Birgittine monastery the Rule should be read aloud once a month when the male and female convents had common meals; see Risberg *Liber usuum*, 'Introduction,' 23.

days. It informs the reader what kind of diet to keep on different fasting days, and thus diet is strongly connected to the liturgical calendar. The Rule is very assertive in differentiating the diet on days of fasting, but rarely calls for fasting on only water and bread. When fasting on only water and bread, the nun must be healthy and not weakened by age, the Rule states. The sick and weak should refrain from fasting until they had recovered. If a sister had been ordered to fast on bread and water as punishment, even she had to be healthy, according to the Rule, so as to be able to fast.[35] Birgitta's Rule thus confirms that nuns should make sure that the body gets what it needs – when nuns fasted, the Rule confirms that they would usually eat other things than meat. They would seldom fast only on water and bread; even if they did, they had to be strong and healthy. Strong and healthy are used synonymously here, which is how Katerina understood the Rule.[36]

I can conclude that for Birgitta the foundation of good health was to eat properly and to eat the right kinds of food, according to the liturgical calendar. From the regulations, it can be deduced that lack of food can endanger a person's health. Thus, no anorectic fasting should take place. This is in line with Musumeci, Threlfall-Holmes, and others regarding the late medieval interpretation of the Rule of Saint Benedict.[37]

Regula Salvatoris informs us not only of diet connected to the liturgical calendar, but of the diet during ordinary weeks as well. The Birgittine Rule explicitly says that a monk or nun could eat meat on four named days in an ordinary week, that is, on Sundays, Mondays, Tuesdays, and Thursdays. Eating that much meat is in line with Johan Söderberg's research on what was eaten at Vadstena monastery. Moreover, Swedish scholars have found that the calorie intake in Swedish monasteries was high, but that the intake of vegetables was too low for a healthy diet.[38]

35 *Regula Salvatoris*, ch. 24, 9, and 18.

36 The opposite is also obvious; when you are sick, you are weak: *Pepper for Prayer*, letters 17 and 26.

37 Musumeci, 'Urban Influence,' 21–22, 33–34; Threlfall-Holmes, *Monks and Markets*, 221. Threlfall-Holmes notes a much higher level of spending on luxurious foodstuffs at Durham than at Westminster, with spending on both wine and spices much higher than at Westminster (222): the monks' standard of dress was much lower than might be suggested by their intake of food and spices. In all, they were not as 'corrupt or luxurious as suggested by post-reformation caricature' (222).

38 *Regula Salvatoris*, ch. 9; Söderberg, 'Oceanic Thirst,' table 4, p. 142; table 5, p. 143; Tollin, 'Medeltida,' 306–309. Compare the same high consumption of meat and low consumption of vegetables at Durham Priory in Threlfall-Holmes, '*Monks and Markets*,' 73–74. Musumeci found that the monastery in Florence he studied bought their vegetables at the market; see 'Urban Influence,' 32.

Markus Lindberg has studied rules regarding food and eating in two Birgittine customaries, one for the female and the other for the male convent in Vadstena monastery. There were only minor differences between them. In these customaries, Lindberg found a specified weekly menu. The amounts of luxurious products were very small and spices such as pepper, mustard, and saffron, as well as figs, were only imported for feasts and holidays or for those who were sick or weak. Wine was only purchased for Communion.[39] In this regard, I would say that these luxurious products were reserved for those who were sick and old, which reflects the perception that these luxury goods had healing properties.

Spices in food

Almost every letter that Katerina wrote to Hans Imhof contained a request to have spices delivered to the monastery. To a large extent, spices went right into their pots. To justify why she needed to order such a large amount of spices, she wrote to Hans: 'When we add spices to a meal, we always need the amount for ninety persons, including the priests and the people on the outside who work for the monastery, so that a little bit doesn't go very far if you want it to taste good.[40]

Large quantities of food were prepared when more people worked on repairs or new construction, thus more purchases of food and spices were required.[41] Katerina was responsible for the purchase of spices. Spices were expensive, and they were considered luxury products. Katarina paid for them out of her own pocket. As an experienced businesswoman, she was price-conscious, and always discussed prices with Hans. If a spice, dried fruit, or sugar had become expensive, she either bought less, or more often abstained from buying them at that moment, waiting for the price to go down.[42] Viewed from a moral perspective, perhaps purchasing spices at cheaper prices consoled her conscience. Or did she buy for a lower price as an old habit, because, she as a former merchant was financially frugal?

39 Lindberg, 'Addiciones,' 184–189. One of the sources he used was *Liber usuum fratrum monasterii Vadstenensis = The customary of the Vadstena Brothers*; see also Carlquist, 'Abbedissan,' 17.

40 *Pepper for Prayer*, 97.

41 *Pepper for Prayer*, 51.

42 *Pepper for Prayer*, 61 sugar; 97 grains of paradise is cheap, 99; Hans should wait for reasonable prices for nutmeg, mace, galangal, ginger and pepper, before sending them; *Pepper for Prayer* 181–183; 175 raisins.

According to the Rule, it was permitted, maybe even desirable, to have spices before the big holidays. The spices that Katerina usually bought, or had sent to her by Hans, were the same for Easter and Christmas. At least a month in advance, she ordered nutmeg, cloves, galangal, and ginger, for example.[43] Saffron is the spice they seemed to want at the convent all year round. Katerina placed the monastery's order for an annual ration in December the year before.[44] The uses of saffron sometimes appear in her letters, in medicinal drinks (addressed later), and in foods. Saffron spiced fish dishes, vegetables, and (most commonly) soups at the monastery. Katerina explained to Hans that everybody felt better after having eaten food spiced with saffron.[45] She did not use words indicating health in her references to food; today we would associate Katerina's use of 'felt better' with 'well-being.' Despite the absence of words related to health regarding food, it seems likely that Katerina equated well-being with health.

It is important to keep in mind that 'cooking and pharmacology were closer during the Middle Ages,' and Katerina really believed that spices added nutrition to the food.[46] When the nuns fasted during Advent until Christmas 1516, she wrote to Hans that the spices in the fish and other dishes made it easier for them to get through the fasting period.[47] Additionally, the very taste of a spice, the flavour, could penetrate the mind and affect the whole body positively, according to Katerina and humoral theory of the period.[48] The perception was that flavours penetrated the body and resulted, according to this way of thinking, in balancing the unbalanced fluids in the body. When body fluids were in balance, the person was healthy.

In general, Katerina only brought up the question of food and drink by necessity when there was a lack of access to supplies due to harvest failures.[49] Even in her first letter to Hans, she wrote that the female convent was not as well supplied with food and drink as the male convent. On the other hand, in the same letter, she assured Hans that she had everything she needed, and that the sisters took care of her needs. In other letters, she expressed her confidence that the Lord would give her and the convent what they

43 *Pepper for Prayer*, 63, 151.

44 *Pepper for Prayer*, 163.

45 *Pepper for Prayer*, 129, 163.

46 *Pepper for Prayer*, 53, quote in Freedman, 'Health, Wellness,' 47.

47 *Pepper for Prayer*, 71.

48 *Pepper for Prayer*, 163.

49 *Pepper for Prayer*, 159: a storm 'destroyed everything'; 181: 'we have nothing to eat until we get the new grain'; 209: severe harvest losses, 263.

required so that they would stay healthy.[50] However, the lack of food could endanger a person's health, which was implied in both Katerina's letters and in *Regula Salvatoris*, as was discussed above. Katerina was of the opinion that the Rule guaranteed the inhabitants in a monastery the meal of the day.[51] In Katarina's letters, I did not find any mention of the renunciation of food and drink, and as I observed earlier, nor was there any renouncement of food in the Birgittine Rule.

Spices in refreshments

Shortly after her entry into the monastery in Maihingen, Katerina offered the female convent a medicinal refreshment, which she used to prescribe for her own family, made of powdered spices mixed with sugar. She informed Hans that the sisters had not had refreshments before, so this was something she introduced. In Katarina's words, this novelty made the sisters 'delighted,' and she thought that 'the weak are given better refreshment and strengthened thereby.'[52] Reasoning that spices would improve the health of the weak and sick brought such purchases in line with the Birgittine Rule.

After the first medicinal drink she prepared in 1516, it is implied in subsequent letters that Katerina offered both convents these kinds of salutary drinks on a regularly basis. These beverages were, called *trisanet*.[53] Those that Katerina made always seems to have contained the ingredient sugar, added with different spices, according to season. Some of the spices used in the monastery's food were also used in the monestary's medicinal drinks, such as nutmeg, cloves, and cinnamon. Katerina explicitly said that she used one of these three spices when she prepared her *trisanet*.[54] But which one, we will never know.

We are also barred from knowing which liquid the sugar and spices were mixed with. Were they mixed with water, ale, beer, or wine? It could have been wine, since this was a common liquid binder in this period, especially for herbal mixtures. Wine or vinegar was the liquid binder in the herbal book that the Vadstena Monastery wrote for one of its sister

50 *Pepper for Prayer*, 49, 123, 135.

51 *Pepper for Prayer*, 215.

52 *Pepper for Prayer*, 49.

53 *Pepper for Prayer*, 234–235, 291.

54 *Pepper for Prayer*, 291.

monasteries, Naantali.[55] Wine, like sugar, was often very expensive. If the spices were not mixed with wine or vinegar, they could just as well have been mixed with beer, and drunk to improve intercessory prayer., This notion is based on Katerina's statement: 'They must drink beer during this time of great singing and reading, and they therefore want to buy spices and food for Lent.'[56] Seldom does Katerina comment on the properties of the spices from a humoral pathological viewpoint; she perhaps takes it for granted that such properties and their effects were widely known. When it comes to beverages, some of them contain spices, such as her medicinal drinks, but when she talks of beer as such, it is again connected to sisters performing prayers better. Wine, on the other hand, is something special. Katerina and the abbess repeatedly claim that wine has health-promoting properties and should be given to the elderly and the sick. I will return to this under the next heading.

Katerina thought of herself as contributing to improving her spiritual sisters' work as intercessors for people outside the convent. One of the editors of Katerina's letters, Volker Schier, has written about some examples of Katerina's way of justifying the import of a highly valued spice, such as saffron. Saffron was a spice with which the monastery had previously been unfamiliar. Katerina said that it had properties that elevated and triggered the mind and helped the sisters perform better when singing.[57] In modern medicine, such qualities have been verified. Saffron has been proven to help depressed people and could also have hallucinogenic effects if taken in sufficient amounts or ingested together with wine.[58] Scholars have even confirmed that not only saffron but also nutmeg and hemp had the same effects. Katerina imported a substantial amount of saffron, and thus Schier has tentatively suggested that the nuns could have been able to use it as a hallucinogen, although we do not know if they did. At the very least, these psychoactive substances helped them perform their task as mediators better, Schier argues. This is what Katerina herself used as justification for her import of these spices and argued that the sisters needed them when, during Lent, they had to sing and pray for hours without rest. Schier even goes further by suggesting that they could have used them to fall into a trance or state of ecstasy, so as to momentarily lose the memory of their pained

55 Larsson, *Millefolium*, 34; see *Naantali herbal book*, 153–162 for mixtures with wine or vinegar (the latter is more common); Gruman Martins, 'Understanding,' 177 on wine; Tuten, 'Care,' 127, 132 on wine/vinegar.

56 *Pepper for Prayer*, 185.

57 Schier et al. 'Introduction,' 15, referring to Schier, 'Probing,' 57–72.

58 Schier, 'Probing,' 63.

bodies. Katerina, however, only says that spices and fruits enhanced their minds and well-being: 'One does need to spice up things a bit, especially when the men and the sisters have to sing and pray a lot, and otherwise they do not have much variety in their diet!'[59]

Wine's healing properties

The Birgittine monastery Maria Mai at Maihingen had the privilege of having vineyards of their own.[60] Certain years, when the harvest was good, both convents could look forward to having wine with food on special occasions.[61] But wine was not the staple beverage in Maria Mai; it was beer, just as in other Birgittine monasteries. To have wine as a staple beverage could then be perceived as luxurious, and seen as indulging in something out of the ordinary. When a wine harvest was bad, Katarina pointed out that it was only the male convent that were given wine with their food, and in addition to the wine the male convent received the usual amount of beer.[62] The female convent, on the other hand, only received wine for the sick and for elderly, weak nuns.[63] Katerina and her convent sisters were surely aware of the beneficial properties wine was supposed to have. According to humoral theory, wine could strengthen a weak body because it warmed the blood. Moreover, the specific disease that wine was supposed to cure was melancholy.[64]

Wine's healing properties may also have been known to Birgitta, who in her *Extravagantes* states that spices and wine should be given to the weak and sick.[65] Yet wine was not mentioned in *Regula Salvatoris*.[66] Lindberg found that the monks in Vadstena only used wine for the communion, as far as we know. When he compared the diet amongst the monks in Vadstena with what they ate and drank at the bishopric of Linköping, Lindberg concluded

59 *Pepper for Prayer*, 135, 137.

60 *Pepper for Prayer*, 267.

61 God 'protected our grape harvest in Würtemberg. And so, by the grace of God, we shall have more wine this year than we have had any other year'; *Pepper for Prayer*, 269.

62 *Pepper for Prayer*, 135, 263. Threlfall-Holmes showed that monks at Durham cathedral drank both wine and beer in an ordinary day; *Monks and Markets*, 68.

63 *Pepper for Prayer*, 143.

64 Boquet and Nagy, *Medieval Sensibilities*, 138–140.

65 Lindberg, 'Addiciones,' 188.

66 The Benedictine Rule, on the other hand, allowed for a reasonable amount of wine to be consumed by the monks. See Threlfall-Holmes, *Monks and Markets*, 68 and 73, where the intake of wine at Durham Cathedral is compared with the intake of wine by monks at Westminster.

that the food and drink at the monastery was much humbler than at the bishopric, where wine was indeed included in the diet.[67]

Another indication of the use of wine in healing illnesses at the Birgittine monestary at Maria Mai can be observed when Katerina explains how the abbess, who was responsible for purchasing this luxury product, had bought overly expensive wine of poor quality. However, this wine was bought for the ill monks and sisters of the monastery, which could be interpreted as meaning that despite the high price, it was worth it and that its health-promoting effect did not diminish, even if it did not taste good.[68] Once again, Katerina argued that the luxury product was purchased to promote health, to enhance the nuns' health or well-being.

Bad fumes, bad smells, and salutary odours

In Katerina's writing, it is obvious that it is the woman's task to take care of the sick and dead, whether she is a housewife or a nun. As a nun, Katerina had been entrusted with taking care of one of the older nuns who had been feeble for a year.[69] The norm of the housewife as a caretaker can be illustrated through Katerina's comments on the sad story of the mother who successfully nursed her ill child but who herself perished. Katerina explains that the mother's tragic death was due to having inhaled a large volume of bad fumes.[70] Katerina also gives enigmatic advice to Hans that she wishes him to pass on to his wife, who had taken care of so many sick family members during the year 1517. Katerina worries that his wife could have been exposed to bad vapours in the rooms of all those sick people she assisted. Katerina is of the opinion that these vapours could cause great illness.[71] This opinion is consistent with humoral theory and such an illness should be counteracted by using an appropriate spice or by being bled, or both. Katerina comes back to this topic several times in her letters. She urges Hans's wife to turn to Uncle Pirckheimer for advice on how to avoid illness when tending to sick persons in their rooms.[72] Pirckheimer could give recommendations on which spices to use to counteract bad air. Another way to get rid of the

67 Lindberg, 'Addiciones,' 187–188. Monks at Durham Cathedral indulged themselves with wine, Threlfall-Holmes concludes; *Monks and Markets*, 73.

68 *Pepper for Prayer*, 143.

69 *Pepper for Prayer*, 169.

70 *Pepper for Prayer*, 119.

71 *Pepper for Prayer*, 109; as mentioned, even in letters 17 and 26.

72 *Pepper for Prayer*, 119.

effects from bad fumes was to avoid them and seek places where the air was fresh. Katerina recommended a visit to Maria Mai: 'We have by the grace of God, fine fresh air out here,' a recommendation she repeated many times.[73] Air quality was one of the external factors that affected health, thus such a recommendation was well in line with humoral theory.

Finally, I will address a specific case where bad fumes were to be combated. Bad fumes undoubtedly could be fought with sweet-smelling scents using aromatic spices, and in this case, Katerina recommended pomander.[74] She describes to Hans that pomander is 'supposed to be good for warding off the bad vapours, and on it (the pomander), in the quill of a feather, are the tau sign[75] and many devotional words.' Here, we see a clear example of the conflation of religion, mysticism, and the medicine of that time, something that many other scholars have also noticed in this period.[76] The overall impression, however, is that Katerina shuttles between the religious perspective on health and her understanding of humours, as an educated tradeswoman of the time would. This is why she has to explain what this pomander contains, so that Hans understands the different ingredients that are supposed to activate healing. The salutary odour he understands, but the holy sign and the devotional words are both mystical and religious references and must be clarified.

Combinations of methods

With the exception of the example above combining religious and humoral methods, I have so far described separately the contexts in which spices were used by Katerina to improve or maintain the nuns' health or well-being. In fact, spice treatments in the monastery were combined with other healing methods and practices. This will be exemplified below.

At the beginning of 1517, Hans became ill, and was bedridden in the spring of the same year. From the time Hans had fallen ill, both the male and the female convent in Maihingen had prayed for his recovery. Praying could be seen as the foremost healing practice in the Middle Ages. Praying was,

73 *Pepper for Prayer*, 109.

74 Usually they used the spice clove. *Pepper for Prayer*, 169.

75 The *Tau cross* is representative of salvation and of life, due in part to its association with the sparing of believers in the Bible. As Tau is the last letter in the Hebrew alphabet, it symbolises the revealed Word of God, its completion and perfection. See https://symbolsage.com/tau-cross-symbol-origins/. Accessed April 2022. My guess is that she meant the Franciscan Tau cross.

76 Dumas, 'L'Ymage,' 143–173; Ritchey and Strocchia, 'Introduction'; Barker and Strocchia, 'Household Medicine.'

however, not enough to help a person heal. Katerina informed Hans that both convents turned to Saint Liborius for help, a practice she described thus: 'they place great hope in the saint.' Nevertheless, the outcome of his health was uncertain and Hans needed to have God's mercy to become well.[77] In the end, recovery was in God's hands.[78] God was the ultimate healer. In addition to these 'religious' methods, Katerina suggested that Hans take an enema treatment, or one of Uncle Pirckheimer's medications. Pirckheimer would have recommended a medicine that was made with a spice, since spices were considered to have a greater effect than an herb. Enemas were a common form of treatment according to humoral pathology.[79] Finally, Katerina concludes her comments on Hans's health by returning to a religious standpoint, namely to 'put matters in the Lord's hands.'[80] I agree with Krötzl who has emphasised that faith is a healing method.[81] Katerina considers faith to be crucial but at the same time she recommends Hans use a humoral pathological method, too. Katerina's advice to Hans: 'Just because our dear Lord has long protected and kept you when you were weak, don't neglect to be bled.'[82]

Moreover, this advice informs us that Katerina was of the opinion that a person should contribute to his or her recovery, using available methods, and not solely having faith in God and relying on his mercy. Bleeding was one of these available methods. This practice, according to Katerina, was especially beneficial for those who were sick and for elderly persons in general. Furthermore, she explains, trying to convince Hans of the benefits of bleeding, to promptly bleed a person inflicted with pestilence successfully worked for those who contracted a headache.[83]

Bleeding could also be used for preventive purposes. According to Katerina, to maintain one's health, one could be bled a few times a year. It seems as if recurring bleeding took place amongst the sisters at Maria Mai.[84] Katerina had no problems with conforming to such a practice. She explains to Hans that even elderly, frail nuns recover and become well again after having been bled. Everybody was bled on the same day and Katerina informs

77 *Pepper for Prayer*, 101: quote at 105.

78 *Pepper for Prayer*, letters 2, 5, 16, 17, 18, 26, and 28.

79 *Pepper for Prayer*, 109.

80 *Pepper for Prayer*, 105.

81 For the conceptualisation of faith as a healing method, see Krötzl, 'Saints,' 260–261.

82 *Pepper for Prayer*, 235.

83 *Pepper for Prayer*, 109.

84 Bloodletting was a common practice in European monasteries. An apothecary would come from the nearest town and bleed everyone at the monastery: see Yearl's article 'Bloodletting.'

her cousin that afterwards she usually offers her colleagues a *trisanet*.[85] Here we see again that Katerina combines two medicinal methods: bleeding and a salutary drink. In these instances, the practices are health-promoting rather than curative.

Nevertheless, only God had the power over life and death. At the beginning of 1518, Hans and his wife lost to pestilence their youngest child, their eight-year-old daughter Magdalena. After this loss, Hans's wife, Katharina Muffel, fell into a depression that lasted several months. When Katerina first heard about the tragic event, she was very caring and comforting to both Katharina and Hans. On a medical level, she recommended him to take a salutary drink. It probably contained spiced wine, since wine in itself was supposed to heal sadness.[86] Katerina consoled him with invoking positive thoughts by saying that his daughter was now in the care of the Lord, that the Lord had 'relieved her of many worries and fears,' and that she now, hopefully, experienced great joy.[87] Together, Hans and Katerina tried to comfort Hans's wife in different ways to bring her out of her depression.[88] Several times, Katerina suggested a visit to the monastery for them both in order to escape the town and for a change of scenery and at the same time they could enjoy some fresh, healing air. Healing air would cure the depression: 'Then your dejection would leave all the more quickly,' wrote Katerina.[89] But Katerina also expressed some irritation when the depression lasted, in her opinion, too long, saying that she 'disapprove[d] of the fact that she [was] still so despondent.' The reason for her disapproval was that the daughter Magdalena had lost her life according to God's will. If God had chosen to take their girl, they should accept and conform to his will, she wrote.[90]

In an earlier letter, Katerina had explained the difference between God taking a life and someone being murdered. A murder took place in anger, disagreement and hatred. Parents of a murdered child have more difficulty with the labour of grief than parents whose child has been taken from them by God, Katerina explained. When the Lord takes a life, he redeems that person from evil, but when a murder is committed, it is an evil act.[91] That is why parents of a murdered child suffer more, Katerina explains to Hans in her letter to him. God's presence and care alleviate grief while fresh air

85 *Pepper for Prayer*, 235.
86 Boquet and Nagy, 'Medieval Sensibilities,' 139.
87 *Pepper for Prayer*, 179, 181.
88 *Pepper for Prayer*, 187, 189, 195, 203. How to fight a depression by breathing fresh air.
89 *Pepper for Prayer*, 189.
90 *Pepper for Prayer*, 179–181, 187.
91 *Pepper for prayer*, 181.

helps the depressed to recover faster. Once again, two different healing methods are intertwined!

Conclusion: wellbeing as health in body and soul

When Katerina described health in a living person, she did not separate body from soul.[92] She uses the idiom 'body and soul' in different settings but seems to imply that a complete human being is composed of both parts. She expresses this conjoined relationship in several ways: that 'divine grace' fell on a person's body and soul, or that God invoked all that was 'useful and good,' 'useful and necessary,' or 'prosperous' for body and soul.[93]

For her, God was the ultimate healer.[94] He had the power to deliver a human from illness by invoking healing and by giving the ill person strength to recover. Prayers offered to God helped a sick person regain health, but God's will or mercy was crucial.[95] As the supreme healer, God had the power to inflict a disease on a person, but that was done with the holy purpose of assisting the salvation of a soul, Katerina explains.[96] Even though she considered God had made a person sick, prayers were read in both convents for improved health. Katerina perceived it as the task of her and her sisters to nevertheless actively contribute to a person's recovery.[97]

Food was strongly connected to health, both in Katerina's writing and in the Birgittine Rule, *Regula Salvatoris*. Neither recommended that anyone abstain from food. A person should eat to prevent illness and to maintain health. Spices in food and drinks enhanced well-being and helped the body and mind to perform under weary and harsh conditions. The earlier ideal of controlling the body had given way to the notion of promoting well-being in the late Middle Ages.

92 Scholars have debated the extent to which people in the Middle Ages drew a sharp line between body and soul. See King, 'Why Isn't the Mind–Body Problem Medieval?,' 187: they did separate body from soul, but, medieval thinkers did not go as far as to separate body from the mind. Boquet and Nagy, *Medieval Sensibilities*, especially chapter 5, gives a complete account of how the idiom has changed since Augustine, by studying them in relation to emotions.

93 *Pepper for Prayer*, 197, 225, 227, 243.

94 In hagiographic sources however, faith in saints as healers are strong. There, saints have different kinds of miraculous healing powers. In miracle collections most of the miracles concern healing. When a cult was established after a saint's death, it could result in creating a healing space around the shrine. See Krötzl, 'Saints,' 255–264; Kandzha, 'Female Saints,' 67–90.

95 *Pepper for Prayer*, 109.

96 *Pepper for Prayer*, 217.

97 *Pepper for Prayer*, 221

According to Katerina, it was not only prayers and faith in God that helped a person to get better. Enemas, bleeding, and the use of spices in food, in beverages, and in pharmaceutical remedies had equivalent effects on a person's health and well-being. The religious and the medicinal methods of securing health were intertwined. Medical treatments alone were not enough to become well. No one was healed without God's grace. No remedy could be taken to become well unless God chose it. Nevertheless, Katerina was of the strong opinion that everyone should uphold his or her health with all available methods, and not leave one's health only in God's hands.

Her contribution to what we today would call well-being was that she added beneficial spices to the food of her sisters and made health-promoting drinks that likewise had beneficial spices as their main ingredients. These same spices were used in beverages, food, and in medication. With regard to their curative and health benefits, Katerina seems to have considered the medicinal effects of using spices in these different ways as equivalent. She possessed knowledge of their health-promoting properties, and she had the right contacts to purchase them for a reasonable price. Throughout her letters, Katerina demonstrates a keen consciousness of cost, always seeking the best price and adapting the amount of spices that she asked Hans or his wife to buy for her.[98] And if the price was too high, she abstained from buying spices, waiting for purchase prices to become cheaper.[99] Spices were bought with the argument that the sisters performed their task as intermediators better, or that the minds of the sisters were elevated, or that spices made them healthier, and even some of the disease symptoms of the sick would disappear, and everybody became more cheerful and felt delighted with the intake of spices.

So, did the sisters at Maria Mai indulge themselves? Did they purchase overly luxurious products that were very expensive? My answer would be no. They avoided gluttony according to the second definition of the sin given by Lagerlund, and they did not transgress the Birgittine Rule, except perhaps for the fact that they drank wine. On the other hand, cultivation of grapes was possible at the latitudes in which they lived, making wine modestly available. Another important factor was that the wine's medicinal properties were more strongly rooted in Katerina's time than in Birgitta's, although Birgitta showed that she was familiar with wine's healing properties in her *Extravagantes*.[100] To be able to offer ill or fragile nuns healing wine, the

98 *Pepper for Prayer*, 97, 99, 175, 235, 243, 291.

99 *Pepper for Prayer*, 163: saffron is going up; 183: no nutmeg.

100 The rise in consumption of wine, sugar and spices in Sweden did not take place until the middle of the sixteenth century: see Söderberg, 'Oceanic Thirst,' 147.

abbess had to pay a high price for the purchase of wine in the years their own grape harvest was diminished or destroyed.

In Maria Mai, bleeding and enemas were practised. When Katerina wrote to her cousin about these practices, she presented these methods as successful. Those who received such treatments became cured or strengthened. When she talked about the spices, on the other hand, they were not as often mentioned for their curative properties. Their healing qualities were obvious to both Hans and Katerina: she did not need to convince Hans, who had worked with spices all his life, about the curative properties of spices. However, Katerina needed to convince him that bleeding was a good thing, because he was afraid and tried to avoid practising it.

When she wrote to Hans about the spices in the food and in the beneficial drinks, she described the nuns' appreciation, and also commented on their health. The spices helped them stay up longer (refrain from sleep), and provided the strength to pray and sing for longer periods, and that they felt stronger, healthier, happier, and clearer in their minds. In short, they felt better in every way. Katerina created well-being in Maria Mai. According to Katerina and contemporary humoral theory, if a person felt well, then her humours were in balance and she was then considered healthy. Well-being and the notion of being healthy went hand in hand.

Bibliography

Printed works

Nadhe(n)dals clost(er)s book. Manuscript in Stockholm, National Library of Sweden, MS A 49. Edited by G. E. Klemming, *Läke- och örteböcker från Sveriges medeltid.* SFSS series 1, no. 26, booklet 84.

Pepper for Prayer: The Correspondence of the Birgittine Nun Katerina Lemmel, 1516–1525. Edited and translated by Volker Schier, Corine Schleif, and Anne Simon. Stockholm: Runica et Mediaevalia, 2019.

Risberg, Sara. *Liber usuum fratrum monasterii Vadstenensis = The Customary of the Vadstena Brothers / A Critical Edition*, with an Introduction by Sara Risberg. Stockholm: Almqvist & Wiksell International, 2003.

Saint Bridget's rule: *Regula Salvatoris*

In Swedish: https://litteraturbanken.se/f%C3%B6rfattare/Birgitta/titlar/HimmelskaUppenbarelserIV/sida/7/faksimil.

Medieval copies in Latin:

https://litteraturbanken.se/f%C3%B6rfattare/Birgitta/titlar/OperaMinora1/sida/111/faksimil?show_search_work&s_query=k%C3%B6tt&s_lbworkid=lb502470&s_mediatype=faksimil&s_word_form_only.
or
http://www.alvin-portal.org/alvin/view.jsf?pid=alvin-record%3A175685&dswid=4885 (in a photocopy of a medieval manuscript in the University library in Uppsala, Codex C 25).

Literature

Barker, Sheila, and Sharon Strocchia. 'Household Medicine for a Renaissance Court: Caterina Sforza's Ricettario Reconsidered.' In *Gender, Health and Healing*, edited by Sara Margaret Ritchey and Sharon T. Strocchia, 139–165. Amsterdam: Amsterdam University Press, 2020.

Barnett, Eleanor. 'Reforming Food and Eating in Protestant England, c. 1560–c. 1640.' *The Historical Journal* 63, no. 3 (2020): 507–527.

Bergqvist, Johanna. *Läkare och läkande: Läkekonstens professionalisering i Sverige under medeltid och renässans.* PhD diss., Lunds universitet, 2013.

Boquet, Damien, and Piroska Nagy. *Medieval Sensibilities: A History of Emotions in the Middle Ages.* Cambridge: Polity Press, 2018.

Bynum, Caroline Walker. *Holy Feast and Holy Fast. The Religious Significance of Food to Medieval Women.* London: University of California Press, 1987.

Carlquist, Jonas. 'Abbedissan lånar böcker.' In *Dicit Scriptura. Studier i C-samlingen tillägnade Monica Hedlund*, edited by Sara Risberg, 11–31. Stockholm: Runica et Mediaevalia, 2006.

Christensen Nugues, Charlotte. 'Skolmedicinen i det medeltida Sverige.' In *Til at Stwdera läkedom*, edited by Gunnar Broberg, 61–77. Stockholm: Sekel förlag, 2010.

Dumas, Geneviève. *Santé et société à Montpellier à la fin du Moyen Âge.* Leiden: Brill, 2014.

Dumas, Geneviève. 'L'Ymage de vie: Un Vade-Mecum pour réaliser la "perfection des imparfaiz."' In *Science et technique au Moyen Âge (XIIe – XVe siècles)*, edited by Joël Chandelier, Catherine Verna, and Nicolas Weill-Parot, 143–173. Paris: Presses universitaires de Vincennes, 2017.

Freedman, Paul. 'Health, Wellness and the Allure of Spices in the Middle Ages.' *Journal of Ethnopharmacology* 167, no. 5 (2015): 47–53.

Freedman, Paul. *Out of the East: Spices and the Medieval Imagination.* New Haven, CT: Yale University Press, 2008.

Gruman Martins, Julia. 'Understanding/Controlling the Female Body in Ten Recipes: Print and the Dissemination of Medical Knowledge about Women in the Early Sixteenth Century.' In *Gender, Health and Healing*, edited by Sara Ritchey and Sharon Strocchia, 167–189. Amsterdam: Amsterdam University Press, 2020.

Kandzha, Iliana. 'Female Saints as Agents of Female Healing. Gendered Practices and Patronage in the Cult of St. Cunigunde.' In *Gender, Health and Healing*, edited by Sara Ritchey and Sharon Strocchia, 67–90. Amsterdam: Amsterdam University Press, 2020.

King, Peter. 'Why Isn't the Mind–Body Problem Medieval?' In *Forming the Mind: Essays on the Internal Senses and the Mind/Body Problem from Avicenna to the Medical Enlightenment*, edited by Henrik Lagerlund, 187–205. Berlin: Springer, 2007.

Krötzl, Christian. 'Saints, Healing and Communities in the later Middle Ages: On Roles and Perception.' In *Infirmity in Antiquity and the Middle Ages* [e-book], edited by Jenni Kuuliala and Christian Krötzl, 255–264. Farnham: Ashgate, 2015.

Lagerlund, Henrik. 'Food Ethics in the Middle Ages.' In *The Oxford Handbook of Food Ethics*, edited by Anne Barnhill, Mark Budolfson, and Tyler Doggett, 759–772. New York: Oxford University Press, 2018.

Larsson, Inger. *Millefolium, rölika, näsegräs. Medeltidens svenska växtvärld i lärd tradition* (Vernacular Plant-Names and Plants in Medieval Sweden). Stockholm: Kungl. Skogs- och Lantbruksakademien, 2010.

Lindberg, Markus. 'The Addiciones Prioris Petri: Rules and Reality.' In *Continuity and Change: Papers from the Birgitta Conference at Dartington 2015*, edited by Elin Andersson, Claes Gejrot, E. A. Jones, and Mia Åkerstam, 184–189. Stockholm: Kungl. Vitterhets historie och antikvitets akademien, 2017.

Musumeci, D. S Salvatore. 'The Urban Influence: Shopping and Consumption at the Florentine Monastery of Santa Trinitá the Mid-Fourteenth Century.' In *Food and Faith in Christian Culture*, edited by Ken Albala and Trudy Eden, 21–40. New York: Columbia University Press, 2011.

Nam, Jong Kuk. 'Medieval European Medicine and Asian Spices.' *Ui sahak* 23, no. 2 (2014): 319–342. https://doi.org/10.13081/kjmh.2014.23.319.

Niiranen, Susanna. 'Medical Knowledge of Mental Disorders and Their Cure in Latin and Vernacular Culture in Later Medieval Europe.' In *Encountering Crises of the Mind. Madness, Culture and Society, 1200s–1900s*, eds. Tuomas Laine-Frigren, Jari Eilola, and Markku Hokkanen, 39–68. Leiden: Brill, 2019.

Niiranen, Susanna. 'Mental Disorders in Remedy Collections: A Comparison of Occitan and Swedish Material.' In *Mental (Dis)Order in Later Medieval Europe*, edited by Sari Katajala-Peltomaa and Susanna Niiranen, 151–176. Leiden: Brill, 2014.

Niiranen, Susanna. 'Sexual Incapacity in Medieval Materia Medica.' In *Infirmity in Antiquity and the Middle Ages* [e-book], edited by Jenni Kuuliala and Christian Krötzl, 223–240. Farnham: Ashgate, 2015.

Ritchey, Sara, and Sharon Strocchia. 'Introduction.' In *Gender, Health and Healing*, edited by Sara Ritchey and Sharon Strocchia, 15–40. Amsterdam: Amsterdam University Press, 2020.

Schier, Volker, Corine Schleif, and Anne Simon. 'Introduction.' In *Pepper for Prayer: The Correspondence of the Birgittine Nun Katerina Lemmel, 1516–1525*, edited and translated by Volker Schier, Corine Schleif, and Anne Simon, 9–45. Stockholm: Runica et Mediaevalia, 2019.

Schier, Volker. 'Probing the Mystery of the Use of Saffron in Medieval Nunneries.' In 'Pleasure and Danger in Perception. The Senses in the Middle Ages and the Renaissance.' Special issue, *The Senses and Society* 5 (2010): 57–72. https://doi.org/10.2752/174589310X12549020528176.

Söderberg, Johan. 'Oceanic Thirst? Food Consumption in Mediaeval Sweden.' *Scandinavian Economic History Review* 63, no. 2 (2015):135–153. http://dx.doi.org/10.1080/03585522.2014.987315.

Threlfall-Holmes, Miranda. *Monks and Markets: Durham Cathedral Priory 1460–1520*. Oxford: Oxford University Press, 2005. https://doi.org/10.1093/acprof:oso/9780199253814.001.0001.

Tollin, Clas. 'Medeltida grönsaksodling.' In *Människan och floran*, edited by Håkan Tunón, Börge Pettersson, and Mattias Iwarsson, 304–310. Stockholm: Wahlström & Widstrand, 2005.

Tuten, Belle S. 'Care of the Breast in the Late Middle Ages.' In *Gender, Health and Healing,* edited by Sara Ritchey and Sharon Strocchia, 119–138. Amsterdam: Amsterdam University Press, 2020.

Uddenberg, Nils. 'Boken, bilden och läkekonsten.' In *Läkekonst. Medicinsk illustrationskonst från medeltid till Lennart Nilsson* (Ars Medica. The Art of Medical Illustration from the Middle Ages to Lennart Nilsson), edited by Ove Hagelin, 7–15. Stockholm: Hagströmerbiblioteket, 2010.

Vandereycken, Walter, and Ron Van Deth. *From Fasting Saints to Anorexic Girls: History of Self-Starvation*. London: Athlone Press, 1993.

Yearl, Mary Katherine Keblinger. 'Bloodletting as Recreation in the Monasteries of Medieval Europe.' In *Between Text and Patient. The Medical Enterprise in Medieval and Early Modern Europe*, edited by Florence Eliza Glaze and Brian K. Nance, ix–570. Micrologus' Library 39. Sismel: Edizioni del Galuzzo, 2011.

About the Author

Gabriela Bjarne Larsson is Reader in History at Stockholm University, author of several books, the latest from 2019. She is currently studying ordinary burgher women's religious activities after the dissolution of the guilds in Stockholm. She has an ongoing project on property relations amongst burghers in sixteenth century Stockholm.

6. Curing Madness and Mental Disturbances: Religious Healing Activities in Early Modern Swedish Local Communities

Riikka Miettinen

Abstract

The chapter discusses how religion and religious practices were used in healing madness in seventeenth- and early eighteenth-century Sweden. According to holistic ideas on health, true faith demonstrated via religious practice was vital both for recovering from illnesses and for upholding and improving one's health. The afflicted themselves, and their kin, as well as parish communities and clergy sought alleviation from mental disturbances through prayer, hymn singing and other religious rituals. These spiritual healing practices that were in line with the era's orthodox Lutheranism were encouraged by medical and church authorities. Local clergy assisted in this process, by counselling, visitations, and organising communal prayers in churches. Families and other local communities could also participate in the healing process.

Keywords: history of madness, history of insanity, religious healing, lived religion, mental health care, early modern Sweden

Introduction

The chapter examines mental health care in early modern Swedish local communities, and in particular the religious activities that were aimed at finding cures for or alleviating madness and mental disturbances. After briefly providing background about the role of religion in medicine and healing in the early modern culture, the chapter discusses the spiritual

---

Eyice, M. and C. Forss (eds.), *Health and Society in Early Modern Sweden*.
Taylor & Francis Group 2024
DOI 10.5117/9789463724296_CH06

healing practices carried out at the local level, in particular by local clergy and the rural lay communities, in early modern Sweden (including Finland) during the seventeenth and early eighteenth centuries (c. 1600s–1730s). This time frame covers the era when the Swedish Realm was at its largest and the period of Lutheran Orthodoxy. This period is characterised as a time when religion was an integral part of medicine. Moreover, this is a time when many new natural-scientific and medical ideas, and the professionalisation and 'secularisation' of medicine, were only slowly contributing to the healing practices in the northern periphery of Europe.[1]

A court record from southwestern Finland from 1700 offers a starting point and a good example about the ways religion, and churchmen, were involved in healthcare. Around the year 1680 Brita, a soldier's widow in her late fifties, lost her mind, or started suffering from an undetermined 'weakness in the head' (Swe. *hufwud swaghet*). This illness was so grave that she had to be kept under constant watch. She was unable to work and support herself, and thus resided in her nephew's household where she received care. Her family decided to turn to the local pastor; Brita was transported to the vicarage where she stayed for some time while the pastor consoled her with 'God's Word' during her extended stay. This, at least according to others, eased her ailment. However, Brita continued to suffer from it for the next twenty years, to the extent that she often went missing in the woods and had to be guarded.[2] This chapter explores why such measures were taken and what other religious means of healing were used in the Swedish local, primarily rural communities. The following discussion focuses on the practical solutions and the types of activities that incorporated Christian religious elements and were aimed at healing or alleviating the condition of being mad or mentally 'ill.'

Various studies have discussed the strong relationship between medicine and religion, and religious forms of healing illnesses, including mental disturbances in early modern Europe, as well as the longevity of these practices.[3] Religious understandings of madness, and discourses in experiencing and expressing mental afflictions, were prevalent in the early modern world.[4]

1 See also the introduction and Hjalmar Fors's and Maria Sjöberg's chapters in this volume.

2 National Archives of Finland (KA): Renoverade domböcker (RT) Ylä-Satakunta KO a 11: 1323–1327, Loimijoki, 7–8 May 1700.

3 For example, Classen, *Mental Health, Spirituality, and Religion*; Duffin, *Medical Miracles*; Grell and Cunningham, eds., *Medicine and the Reformation*; Hayward, 'Psychiatry and Religion'; Joutsivuo, 'Ruumiin vai sielun hoitoa'; Lederer, 'Psychiatry in the Sixteenth Century?'; Wear, 'Religious Beliefs and Medicine'; Weatherhead, *Psychology, Religion and Healing*.

4 For example, Eilola, 'Defining and Treating Madness,' 79; Eriksson, *Vägen till centralhospitalet*, 35–92; Hodgkin, *Madness in Seventeenth-Century Autobiography*; Lederer, *Madness, Religion and*

Healing activities that incorporated religious elements were one aspect of lived religion, that is, the ways in which religion was 'lived out,' performed and deployed to solve problems in daily life.[5] Beliefs related to mental disturbances, health, and the appropriate means of healing and recovery influenced the lives of the mentally disturbed and their surrounding communities. The chapter shows how religion provided not only culturally and socially acceptable ways to alleviate impairments but also by which means the local communities participated in the healing process.

In standard histories of psychiatry, insanity, and medicine, the focus has typically been on learned medicine, hospitals, and asylums, and measures taken by doctors while the 'lay' and spiritual forms of care have been relatively overlooked. Many historians have criticised the overemphasis on scholarly medicine and institutions, and highlighted the blend of medical-scientific, magical, and religious therapies that were practised in healing and healthcare.[6] The suggested decline of spiritual healing and magic, and the rise of more 'secular' medicine[7] was not dramatic nor clear-cut during the early modern period. Instead, religion, including spiritual treatments and cures, continued to be significant in the 'healthcare market,' characterised by medical pluralism.[8]

This chapter continues the on-going critical discussion by shedding light on the significance of religious practices in healing 'mental' impairments at the local level in early modern Sweden. Other studies have already discussed some aspects of these issues,[9] but with less focus on the spiritual healing activities carried out in the most typical living surroundings, namely rural villages, peasant homes, and parish churches. The vast majority (90–95 per cent) of the early modern Swedish population consisted of rural peasantry. In the large and relatively sparsely populated Swedish Realm, only a small fraction of the 'insane' were confined in hospitals or other poor relief institutions

the State; MacDonald, *Mystical Bedlam*. For continuations in religious discourses of madness, see, e.g., Peschier, *Lost Souls*.

5 About lived religion, see Katajala-Peltomaa, *Demonic Possession*, 2–3; Katajala-Peltomaa and Toivo, 'Religion as Experience'; Katajala-Peltomaa and Toivo, 'Introduction: Religion,' 1–5.

6 E.g., Harley, 'Spiritual Physic'; Lederer, *Madness, Religion and the State*; MacDonald, *Mystical Bedlam*; MacDonald, 'Religion, Social Change'; Mellyn, 'Healers and Healing.'

7 E.g., Mortimer, *The Dying*; Thomas, *Religion and the Decline of Magic*.

8 E.g., Cunningham and Grell, eds., *Religio Medici*; Grell and Cunningham, *Medicine and Religion*; Gentilcore, *Healers and Healing*, see especially ch. 6 and 7; Houston, *Madness and Society*, 293–330; Lindemann, *Medicine and Society*, 75–77, 231, 254–256; Mellyn, 'Healers and Healing'; Stolberg, *Experiencing Illness*.

9 Esp. Eriksson, *Vägen till centralhospitalet*, esp. 35–92; and Eilola, 'Defining and Treating Madness.'

that were few and far between. During the historical period in question, educated physicians, apothecaries, and chemical substances were mostly available for the wealthier, higher estates and in major towns. Thus, the care and attempts at healing took generally place at the local scene. Like elsewhere in early modern Europe,[10] the main providers of mental health care (to use a modern term) in the Nordic countries were the kin of the afflicted, their local communities, and the clergy. The mentally disturbed were typically members of several local communities, such as farms and households, kin groups, work communities, and parish congregations.

It must be pointed out that there were some cultural and regional differences in the vast Realm, some of which might have significance regarding healing practices. For example, the regions of central Sweden and western Finland were more populous and well connected to central institutional organisations, including universities and ecclesiastical authorities that may have influenced the practices. In turn, northern and eastern parts of the Realm were peripheral and forested areas with people living in tiny hamlets. The culture, languages, and religions practised in the easternmost regions, especially in the Kexholm and Karelian areas, and the Sámi regions in the north, differed to some extent from the rest. However, the Lutheran religion and Church had widely established its foothold, and the cases discussed here come from the more fully integrated and acculturated regions.[11]

Madness and insanity are used as vague umbrella terms here, encompassing different types of illnesses, impairments, and disturbances that were understood as having mental manifestations. People of this period did distinguish between conditions, such as impairments and disorders, that had mental manifestations. 'Mental' illnesses were ultimately manifestations of bodily, humoral disruptions that affected rational faculties and functions, behaviour and feelings, as well as symptoms appearing elsewhere in the body. They could be conditions that contemporaries considered as madness, or as long- or short-term illnesses and disturbances that affected the reason and mental capacities of the person.[12] These conditions signalled various

10 E.g., Houston, *Madness and Society*, 315, passim; Mellyn, 'Healers and Healing,' esp. 85–86; Thomas, *Religion and the Decline of Magic*, 18.

11 Miettinen, *Suicide, Law, and Community*, 3–5, 16–17.

12 Madness is used here, alongside insanity and mental disturbances, as umbrella terms referring to conditions that were considered pathological and affecting the 'mind' in early modern Sweden. It must be emphasised that these concepts are too vague and all-encompassing to aptly describe all the variations of 'mental' disorders and afflictions that the early modern people spoke about. See also Lederer, *Madness, Religion and the State*, 154–158; and Mellyn, *Mad Tuscans*, 19. The early modern Swedish vocabulary referring to disordered minds was rich and

types of 'weaknesses in the head' (Swe. *hufwud swaghet*) that were at the time considered pathological and required healing intervention. The 'mad' or mentally disturbed were those whose thoughts, feelings, and actions seemed unreasonable to others.

However, ultimately, the division between 'mental' and bodily impairments is as blurred as is the distinction between religious cures and other healing interventions. In early modern culture, the (health of the) body, mind, and soul, and the physical and spiritual cures of illnesses, were interrelated and entangled. Although 'natural' and physical remedies, such as plant extracts and dietary prescriptions, were distinguished from spiritual and 'supernatural' restoratives, their healing powers and the person's recovery nonetheless depended on God and required faith.[13] On the one hand, virtually all religious practice carried out while a person was 'ill' can be understood in the realm of healing and alleviation – after all, performing one's faith in all acceptable ways was essential for recovery. On the other hand, 'spiritual physic'[14] was practised for troubled souls in general, for example for those not (yet) 'ill' or mad but despairing or suffering other spiritual afflictions. Moreover, religious practice was crucial not only for restoring health but also for keeping a person healthy,[15] as well as for preparing for a person's death.

In what follows, I will focus on religious activities that are mentioned as intended specifically to heal or alleviate 'mental' impairments. I will also examine the out-of-the-ordinary religious practice by, or directed to, those who were not considered to be dying but who were described in terms that referred to conditions that disordered the 'mind.' It must be noted that some of these practices could include magical elements and religious rituals that were disapproved of and considered illicit. Religion and magic were intertwined and the boundaries between them blurred and porous. Consequently, people and authorities negotiated the limits of

is difficult to translate into English, including e.g., *hufwudswaghet* ('weakness in the head'); *hufwudswag* and *sinnesswag* ('weak in the head/mind'); *galen*(*skap*) and *dår*(*skap/het*), *tokig* (mad, lunatic); *afwita* and *ursinnig* ('out of one's senses'); *fåna/fånig* (crazy, half-witted, fool); *förwirrat* (confused, 'dizzy' in the head); *besatt*(*het*) (mad, possessed); *intet wid sitt förstånd, intet wid sina fulla sinnen* (not in one's right mind), and terms for specific illnesses such as *melancholia*, *mania*, *furor*/*raseri*. There was no specific distinction between intellectual or cognitive disabilities and insanity in the terminology.

13 Lindemann, *Medicine and Society*, 59, 255–256, passim; Mellyn, 'Healers and Healing,' 88–95; Ross, *Care of Bodies*, esp. 272–288, 367–375.

14 Lederer, 'Psychiatry in the Sixteenth Century?'; Lederer, *Madness, Religion and the State*, 1, passim; MacDonald, *Mystical Bedlam*, 217–231.

15 See also Kassell and Ralley, 'Prayer and Physic.'

what was approved and in line with the era's orthodox Lutheran thinking on a case-by-case basis.[16]

The study's material consists of case descriptions and instructions involving healing mental disturbances and the 'mad' through religion, which have been found in various types of sources including court records and other judicial documents, journals, and a selection of printed medical treatises, advice manuals, and Lutheran clerical guidelines. Rather than relying on scholarly medical and theological treatises, the emphasis is on sources that mention activities carried out and practised in local, primarily rural communities. Although the focus is on the typical rural village and parish communities, we can assume that similar practices were also used in towns. After all, the medical and clerical advice, at least in the printed treatises, was the same, and it is likely that at least the more religious town dwellers subscribed to the recommended spiritual healing methods, even if they had greater access to town doctors and apothecaries.

It must be noted that the primary material includes no ego-documents by the mentally afflicted themselves – such documents are rarely available from this time and region. However, supplementary material is also used from a slightly later period. The notes of a provincial doctor, active in northern Sweden in the mid-eighteenth century (Nils Gissler, 1715–1771) are part of the material examined.[17] Typically, the available sources present the mentally disturbed as the objects of some measures and interventions rather than as active agents who, for example, write about their own experiences and personal activities aimed at recovery. Nevertheless, even the more official, judicial, and administrative documents now and then describe – at times in detail – the everyday lives and care of the afflicted. Many types of sources, such as court records and medical treatises, describe their interactions with other people and activities related to healing. For example, some of the rare, preserved journals written by clergy and others include references to encounters and spiritual therapies with the 'mad' and afflicted. However, the descriptions of religious healing in the available sources are oftentimes brief, and the activities mentioned only in passing – which itself suggests that acts of religious healing were so ordinary and commonplace that they did not deserve special attention and documentation.

16 See also Toivo, *Faith and Magic* and De Waardt, 'Chasing Demons,' esp. 173–174.

17 Gissler, *Några minnets qwarlefwor*. Gissler (1715–1771) most likely made his notes in the 1750s and 1760s. Many thanks to Jonas Liliequist for providing the transcription of this source.

Healthy 'minds' and the significance of faith and religious practice

Like other European medical and humoral thinking of the time, the Swedish printed medical treatises and advice manuals are characterised by holistic ideas of health (Swe. *hälsa, sundheet*): the body, mind, and soul are in constant, intimate interaction, and their unified condition generates well-being, or the 'good health' or 'ill-health' of a person. Inflictions on the body or the soul that arise from anywhere in the material or supernatural worlds, such as the environment, movements of celestial objects, the Devil or one's diet, sin or religious practice, could harm the person's humoral balance and thus health. Everything is interconnected; thus the material body pesters the soul, and one's senses, rational capacities and 'mind' (Swe. *sinne*)[18] are affected by the body's humoral constitution. Passions can be harmful but also beneficial for one's health. The condition of one's soul (Swe. *siälen*), as a distinct entity, was an integral part of this whole, and its state could predispose and expose one's body to certain illnesses.[19]

A person was healthy when he could, 'in the right way and without fault,' carry out his tasks 'as should naturally take place.'[20] Most importantly, 'good health' entailed the ability to work and the absence of illness and other 'faults' (Swe. *fel*).[21] Mental and behavioural capacities, such as the ability to reason and speak sensibly, were also involved. Maintaining a steady, calm (Swe. *stadig, still*) temperament, 'mind' and mood was important, as was the moderation of one's affects and passions as well as overcoming certain negative passions. Calmness, cheerfulness, and sociability were signs of good health and considered vital for maintaining it. Excessive affects and passions, which manifested themselves in erratic and disorderly behaviour, were signs of illness and imbalanced or impure humoral constitutions.[22] Like the boundaries between bodies, minds, and souls, the use of terms

18 Cf. *Svenska Akademiens Ordbok* (*SAOB*): *sinne. Sinne* had various connotations in early modern Swedish, including sense, mind, and condition of the soul. Its use in the printed medical literature is ambiguous.

19 E.g., Sparman, *Sundhetzens speghel*, passim, e.g., 137. See also Joutsivuo, 'Ruumiin vai sielun hoitoa,' esp. 76–79. For these ideas in early modern European medicine, see, e.g., Lederer, *Madness, Religion and the State*, 31–35; Lindemann, *Medicine and Society*, 13–16.

20 Sparman, *Sundhetzens speghel*, Förtaal om Sundhetzens natur, n.p.

21 See also Anton Runesson's chapter in this volume.

22 E.g., Sparman, *Sundhetzens speghel*, passim, e.g., Förtaal om Sundhetzens natur, and 140–191. On the importance of managing and moderating one's passions and keeping them in one's power for not being like 'a wild beast,' see, e.g., De Britaine, *Klokhets och skyldighets reglor*, esp. 95–108.

referring to minds, souls, moods, and tempers was blurred and their connotations ambiguous.[23]

Several illnesses had symptoms that affected mental capacities or could manifest themselves in 'moods' and behaviours that hampered daily life. Medical advice books, intended for the peasantry, describe various complex conditions that incapacitated one's sense or reason (Swe. *förnufftet*), including specific 'illnesses of the head,' such as mania (Swe. *mania*, people who were *wild*), raving madness (Swe. *raseri, rasande*), fevers and falling sickness. Though not necessarily considered 'full' madness, the described illnesses were understood as (mental) disturbances that were pathological and required healing activities. They occurred on a wide spectrum and could be episodic. In other words, mental health or 'ill-health' was not perceived as binary – instead, madness, or disordered minds, occurred on a sliding scale. For example, 'weaknesses in the head' (Swe. *hufwud swaghet*) could appear in different degrees, completely disabling a person or less drastically affecting people's rational faculties and moods. *Melancholia* was an illness that had diverse bodily, behavioural, and emotional symptoms, most predominantly overbearing sadness and gloominess. At times, it was called 'gloom-mindedness' (Swe. *Swårmodighet*), although a person could also be gloomy and melancholic by constitution or more temporary, for example, due to 'natural' passions.[24] Accompanying phrases and descriptions of behaviours show when this condition was regarded as madness and an ailment. The signs of madness and mental illness included out-of-the-ordinary, disorderly behaviours such as delusional or otherwise irrational lines of reasoning and speech, excessive, immoderate feelings and their expressions, chronic or temporary inability to work, and, at worst, erratic violence.[25]

As the condition of the soul was integral to health and well-being, tending to the soul via faith and religious practice was crucial. Maintaining and restoring the balance of the soul was also part of the 'spiritual physic' that the clergy provided for those suffering from all sorts of afflictions, ranging from feelings of anxiety and of fear to despair, madness, and demonic temptations and possession. The Christian sacraments, prayer, and spiritual consolation were thought to help those considered mad, otherwise ill, or aid the sane but troubled and afflicted due to despair, compunctions, doubts, fears, or evil

23 Cf. *Svenska Akademiens Ordbok* (*SAOB*): *sinne, själ, mod, temperament.* Likewise, words referring to feeling and emotion are difficult to translate and their use is mixed (e.g., *känna, affect, passion, sinnetz rörelser*).

24 E.g., Colerus, *Oeconomia*; Lindh, *Huusz-apoteek*; Olai, *Een Nyttigh Läkere Book*; Sparman, *Sundhetzens speghel.*

25 Eilola, 'Defining and Treating Madness'; Miettinen, *Suicide, Law, and Community*, 207–215.

thoughts.[26] Offering solace and spiritual guidance for the mentally afflicted, anxious and despaired had long been considered a central task of the local clergy. Many Lutheran manuals for the clergy had specific guidelines on how to console the spiritually anxious and despairing, and several early modern Nordic theologians and other writers wrote extensively about this topic.[27] It is somewhat anachronistic to try to distinguish spiritual healing activities from spiritual physic, as both were practised to uphold and improve health and cure 'ill' conditions.

Various Swedish medical treatises and advice books of the time emphasise how true faith and trust in God are pivotal for healing. Even if more 'natural' cures were recommended, recovery ultimately depended on God.[28] This can be seen, for example, in the medical treatises about the use and healing powers of mineral wells and waters, which were published in abundance in Sweden. Not only did the waters receive their beneficial capacities from God, but their curative force and the patient's recovery ultimately rested in God's hands, as noted in the medical treatises.[29] However, faith alone was not enough. For medicine and healing to be effective, demonstrating one's faith via religious practice, especially prayer, was also emphasised in Protestant and Lutheran thinking.[30] Alongside prayer, confession and true repentance of sins, followed by partaking in Holy Communion, would remove the sin and 'purify' the soul, and thus aid in healing.[31]

The significance of faith and religious practice is also connected to the notion that the Devil could cause illness and disturbances. This aetiology of illnesses was widely accepted especially before the eighteenth century.[32] Some believed that the Devil could even possess and make people mad. For example, Olof Broman, an active priest from 1710 until the 1740s, mentioned

26 Lederer, 'Psychiatry in the Sixteenth Century?'; Lederer, *Madness, Religion and the State*, 1, 6–8, passim; MacDonald, *Mystical Bedlam*, 217–231.

27 E.g., Church Law of 1686, Cap. XVII: Om Siukas och Fångars Besökning, esp. § IX; *Handbok* 1693, esp. 143–149. 'Self-help' guidance and instructions on how to help those who suffer from melancholia, compunctions/bad conscience, sadness, impatience, fear of death, bad thoughts, etc., are found in Balduin, *Samwetz plåster*, 9–93. See also, e.g., Hemmingsen, *Antidotum*.

28 E.g., Hjärne, *Een uthförlig Berättelse*; Lindh, *Huusz-apoteek*.

29 E.g., Hjärne, *Een uthförlig Berättelse*; Tranaeus, *Medewij suurbrunnars*.

30 E.g., Grell, 'Caspar Bartholin,' esp. 78–79; Kassell and Ralley, 'Prayer and Physic'; Ross, *Care of Bodies*, esp. 376–387; Wear, 'Puritan Perceptions of Illness,' 60–61, 73–74; Wear, 'Religious Beliefs and Medicine,' esp. 153. About the importance of faith and prayer for healing in the Middle Ages and in the sixteenth century, see Gabriela Bjarne Larsson's chapter in this volume.

31 E.g., Balduin, *Samwetz plåster*. In early modern England, see Newton, *Misery to Mirth*, 135–137.

32 Eilola, 'Defining and Treating Madness,' 78, 85; Eriksson, *Vägen till centralhospitalet*, 74–87; Sandholm, *Kyrkan och hospitalshjonen*, 242–245. On the Devil causing melancholia, see, e.g., Balduin, *Samwetz plåster*, 12–13.

that he had encountered two or three persons who had been possessed by the Devil.[33] A treatise from 1744, describing the use of Camphor in treating mania, mentions that such beliefs were still widespread among the common folk in Sweden; they believed that the 'unfortunate people' who suffered from mania are beset, or possessed by the evil spirit.[34] Religious rituals were considered the best cures for illnesses and disturbances connected to supernatural causes, such as the Devil or witchcraft. Moreover, it was believed that diligent religious practice and good knowledge of the scriptures would serve as protection against the Devil, and thus, could in part prevent ailments.[35]

The role of the local clergy in healing madness and mental disturbances

Although certain healing activities and rituals – such as praying to saints and relics, conducting pilgrimages, taking part in most Church processions, and exorcism rituals that clerics mediated – were refused after the Reformation, the Protestant clergy continued to have a significant role in the healing process, albeit diminished in comparison to their Catholic counterparts. Even if their power of, or intercession in, healing had been stripped down, Protestant clergymen still had the important task of offering pastoral counselling and religious guidance and assisting the faith and piety of the ill.[36] Ministers and other clergymen of all sects were involved in diverse spiritual healing activities. In the Protestant world, this comprised most importantly visitations, prayer, and spiritual consolation for the ill, including the mad.[37]

Visitations and communions for the sick continued to be an important pastoral duty also in Lutheran Sweden. These activities were regulated, and the clergy were instructed about them in many pastoral manuals and ecclesiastical guidelines. Pastors were expected to make visitations (Swe. *sockenbud*) and provide pastoral services and consolation at the homes of

33 Eriksson, *Vägen till centralhospitalet*, 84.

34 Triewald, *Rön angående Camphers*, 57.

35 Eilola, 'Defining and Treating Madness,' esp. 80; Manninen, 'Ylioppilas parantajana,' 88.

36 Lindemann, *Medicine and Society*, 254–256.

37 E.g., Eriksson, *Vägen till centralhospitalet*, 53–56; Harley, 'Spiritual Physic'; Houston, *Madness and Society*, 314–316; Jimenez, *Changing Faces of Madness*, 44–45; MacDonald, *Mystical Bedlam*, 8, 226–229; Schmidt, *Melancholy*, esp. 77–82; de Waardt, 'Chasing demons.'

the ill, and for those institutionalised at hospitals and poorhouses.[38] In part, this had to do with the ideals and preparations for a 'good death,' in particular promoting the importance of true faith and repentance.[39] But the services provided by the clergy also entailed a restorative function: they were not only carried out for those who were considered to be dying. The word of God and the sacraments that the pastor offered were considered to be 'of use,' supplying the ill 'better strength and state of being, both in the body and the soul.' This is also why the local clergy was to be hastily contacted if someone showed signs of illness: the more time the pastor had with the ill person, the better.[40]

At least some of the local clergy followed the ecclesiastical guidelines and either visited the homes of the mentally disturbed or received visits from them, consoling and – a common phrase – 'strengthening them with the words of God.'[41] We can assume that there were individual and regional differences in this practice, depending on, for example, personal motivations of clergymen, distances between destinations, as well as travel and weather conditions. It is also possible that the visitations and personal services were more likely provided for those who had an established position in the parish, for example for the members of landholding peasant kin groups who, over several generations, had had farms in the near vicinity. However, as the case material here has not been collected systematically and comes from different parts of the Swedish Realm over a long period of time, it is difficult to say much about the social and regional differences.

To give an example, pastor Petrus Magni Gyllenius (1622–1675), who recorded his travels and tasks in his journal, mentions some of these encounters in southwestern Sweden in the 1660s. He had visited an elderly woman who was 'beset' or mad (Swe. *besatt*) and tormented by the 'bad spirit,' having had the same illness (Swe. *siukdom*) since her youth. When she had an attack,

38 E.g., Church Law of 1686, Cap. XVII: Om Siukas och Fångars Besökning, and Cap. XXVIII: Om Hospitaler, esp. § X; *Handbok* 1693, 125–149; Sandholm, *Kyrkan och hospitalshjonen*, 382–394; Sundmark, *Sjukbesök*. For pastoral duties and services and religious practice in early modern hospitals and poorhouses, see Annola and Miettinen, 'Piety and Prayers,' esp. 135–140.

39 About the ideal preparations for death, see, e.g., Balduin, *Samwetz plåster*, esp. 50–65.

40 Church Law of 1686, Cap. XVII: § III.

41 E.g., Riksarkivet (RA): Svea Hovrätt Advokatfiskalens arkiv: Collections of Renoverade domböcker (SHA): Kopparbergs län 23b: 892–899, Husby, 14 February 1687; Upplands län 53b: 556v–561v, Lagunda, 20 November 1691; and Kopparbergs län 30a: 560–562, Sundborn, 22 May 1694. See also KA: RT Turku Town court RO z 34: 119–123, Turku 7 April 1666; Ylä-Satakunta KO a 11: 1323–1327, Loimijoki, 7–8 May 1700; and Etelä-Pohjanmaa KO a: 20: 1184–1185, Ilmajoki, 17 May 1702. Many cases in which the local clergy visited the 'mad' patients of doctor Nils Gissler in Nothern Sweden in the 1750s and 1760s are described in Gissler, *Några minnets qwarlefwor*.

she had to be held down by ten men, but when she was calm, the pastor could read prayers to her, and 'consoled her with the words of God.'[42] He was also called into the home of a rural constable (Swe. *länsman*) to console a wife who had 'gloomy thoughts and a guilty conscience' and was weak and restless, at times unable to sleep at night. He visited the woman every day once or twice for several weeks until she got better – which was, according to the pastor, a timely cure sent by God.[43]

Some of the mentally disturbed required repeated visits, even for months on end. For example, in 1695 a peasant wife named Anna, demanded a great deal of attention from the local clergy. She was described as a highly devout woman who suffered from major 'weakness in the head' (Swe. *hufwud-swaghet*). The pastor visited her on several occasions and consoled her both at her home and in the vicarage.[44] The participation of the local clergy comes across vividly in many suicide cases involving those considered insane. The local pastors and chaplains are mentioned as common guests at the homes, offering counselling and 'God's word' for the ill.[45]

It is noteworthy that the clergy appear to have been particularly involved with people suffering from illnesses and disturbances that were attributed to spiritual or supernatural causes, and in cases of melancholia.[46] Naturally, ailments that were thought to be caused by devilish forces, witchcraft, or personal sin could be best overcome or alleviated by turning to God and to the specialists of true faith and suitable religious practice and rituals. Melancholia resembled and typically manifested itself in similar ways to grief, despair, and doubt. Alongside the cardinal symptom of great sorrow, this ailment often entailed 'deviant' spirituality and susceptibility to thoughts, illusions and hallucinations sent by the Devil. The treatment of all these conditions belonged to the expertise of the clergy.[47] This speciality comes across, for example, in a case from Sundborn, central Sweden. The

42 Gyllenius, *Diarum Gyllenianum*, 246.

43 Gyllenius, *Diarum Gyllenianum*, 316–317. Many thanks to Annika Sandén for these excerpts.

44 RA: SHA Gävleborgs län 45a: 80v–82v, Forsa, Idenor, Hög, Rogsta, Illsbo, and Tuna, n.d. 1695.

45 Miettinen, *Suicide, Law, and Community*, esp. 180, 206. Also, if the kin or household had not called for clergy to the scene when someone had shown signs of madness or mental afflictions, the households were at times questioned about why they had not done this duty and could be reprimanded for such negligence. E.g., KA: RT Northern Ostrobothnia KO a 3:162–63, Liminka, 9–12 February 1683.

46 See also Lindemann, *Medicine and Society*, 15; Mellyn, 'Healers and Healing,' 93–95; in treating melancholia in eighteenth-century England, see Ingram, 'Deciphering Difference,' 189–192.

47 MacDonald, *Mystical Bedlam*, 153–158, 218–229; Miettinen, 'Constructing "Mad" Religious Experiences,' esp. 182; Schmidt, *Melancholy*, esp. 49–64.

court records from 1694 mention how the late parish pastor had suffered from heavy melancholia but had ultimately been able to overcome it, as he, as a 'learned clergyman,' could both be consoled by others and spiritually console himself. This ailment ran in the family. The pastor's daughter also suffered from it throughout her life and was treated by her husband, a pastor.[48] Thus, it is likely that people suffering from certain types of madness were thought to deserve more clerical attention.

Descriptions of the 'spiritual therapies' and about what the clergy did and said, are vague. Besides the Lord's prayer, the clergy read unspecified prayers and biblical passages and sang hymns with the afflicted. The clergy also encouraged repentance, provided religious instruction, and advised personal religious practice. During visitations, they could also listen to the person's confessed sins and give Holy Communion, at least when the mad person was having a lucid moment.[49] The clergy took advice from clerical guidelines and devotional literature. For example, the clerical handbook of 1693 includes several phrases, questions, and words of comfort as well as specific prayers to console and strengthen the faith of the 'ill' whom they visited.[50] Even if the confession of sins was done in private, as instructed in ecclesiastical guidelines, other household members could participate in the prayer and spiritual activities at the homes. For example, in 1686 the local pastor and chaplain visited Karin, a peasant's wife, who was greatly troubled and suffering from 'mental weakness' (Swe. *sinnes swagheet*) and melancholia. The chaplain described how he had read many prayers and sang hymns with Karin, and repeatedly read the Lord's prayer with her, during which she had squeezed the hand of the chaplain's wife so tightly that it hurt the rest of the day.[51]

Another way that the local clergy took part in treating the mad and other 'ill' was to organise public, joint prayers in the church.[52] This also

48 RA: SHA Kopparbergs län 30a: 560–562, Sundborn, 22 May 1694.

49 The Church Law of 1686 stated that the insane or half-witted (Swe. *Fånar*) and those with 'mental weakness' should not be let into confession and communion until they come to their senses. Church Law of 1686, Cap. VIII: § III and Cap. XVII: § V.

50 *Handbok* 1693, 125–149. See also Sandholm, *Kyrkan och hospitalshjonen*, 389–394. Daily personal prayer, repentance and asking God's mercy and forgiveness for one's sins were also encouraged. For consoling passages from the Bible and biblical examples, see Balduin, *Samwetz plåster*.

51 RA: SHA Kopparbergs län 23b: 892–899, Husby, 14 February 1687.

52 E.g., Provincial Archives of Uppsala (ULA): Uppsala länsstyrelsens arkiv, Landskansliet D II: 2, Svartlösa, 6 December 1682: since a 'hufwudswagh' man could not dress himself, cried, etc., he was prayed for in the church. KA: RT Kymenkartano län KO a 2: 360v–361, Vehkalahti, 25 November 1672: the clergy said prayers in the pulpit on behalf of a local 'hufwudswagh' man;

allowed the parish members to participate in the healing. For example, the above-mentioned peasant wives, Anna and Karin, were prayed for in the church for several weeks. The local pastor led the prayer from the pulpit, praying for 'God to help and strengthen' Anna, during or after every sermon for over a month.[53] As this practice was written about in such a routine way, only mentioning it in passing, one can assume that it was commonplace for the local clergy and the congregations to pray for the ill parish members at church.

Religious healing activities in the local communities

Very few preserved documents discuss the religious healing practised in local communities specifically or at length; rather, they are mentioned in passing while other matters, such as crimes or disputes involving the mentally disturbed, are at the forefront. However, some of these references not only provide information about the activities but also suggest their prevalence.

Alongside the local clergy, the ill and afflicted had roles in their own healing process. The mad practised personal prayer, churchgoing, repentance, and communions, and other religious activities, such as hymn singing, reading the Bible or reciting passages, to alleviate their conditions. After all, potential healing was contingent on complete and total faith in God, and obedience to Church teachings. Indeed, some of the mentally disturbed were highly involved, even obsessed, with fervent religious practice – desperately seeking divine cure for their condition.[54] Immersion in religious practice could be interpreted by others in many ways. It could be considered as the appropriate, conventional means for healing and reaching 'sanity,' but it

KA: RT Jääski, Lappee, Ranta and Äyräpää KO a 17:235–237, Lappee, 30 September 1680; RA: SHA Kopparbergs län 23b: 892–899, Husby, 14 February 1687; KA: RT Ylä-Satakunta KO a 73: 19v, Orivesi and Kuorevesi, 16–20 January 1753; ULA: Örebro länsstyrelsens arkiv, Landskansliet. D I qa: 3, Glanshammar, 17 July 1686. Also, among other Protestants, Puritans organised joint prayers as part of the communal healing of an individual's illness. Wear, 'Puritan Perceptions of Illness,' 74.

53 RA: SHA Kopparbergs län 23b: 892–899, Husby, 14 February 1687; RA: SHA Gävleborgs län 45a: 80v–82v, Forsa, Idenor, Hög, Rogsta, Illsbo and Tuna, n.d. 1695.

54 E.g., RA: SHA Kopparbergs län 23b: 892–899, Husby, 14 February 1687; ULA: Kopparberg läns häradsrätts arkiv, Serie X, A I: 1, 109–109v, Tuna, 23 September 1689; RA: SHA Gävleborgs län 45a: 80v–82v, Forsa, Idenor, Hög, Rogsta, Illsbo, and Tuna, n.d. 1695; RA: SHA Upplands län 53b: 556v–561v, Lagunda, 20 November 1691.

might also be regarded as a sign of madness, such as religious melancholia, or over-zealous religious enthusiasm.[55]

Surrounding community members also took part in and contributed to the spiritual healing activities. As shown in the previous case examples, others could join the prayers at church or during the pastoral visitations. They could also pray for alleviation and recovery for their kin or friend more privately at home or elsewhere. Although the available cases rarely specify who was involved in the praying, one can assume that it was not only the families and household members of the mad and ill who joined the prayers, but also their village neighbours and friends, and, in the churches, all the attending congregation members.

Prayer was considered particularly potent for treating the mad. For example, in 1730 in Kajaani, a small inland town in northeastern Finland, a young student, Johan Svahn, took upon himself to try to heal a mad, raging woman, who was considered possessed. Brita, the wife of a carpenter, felt herself beset by the devil, raging and delirious. Johan tried to get her to repeat the Lord's prayer and say the name of Jesus. Later, he was sued for beating and whipping Brita while carrying out this 'treatment.' Johan explained that he was acting with good intentions, trying to get Brita to pray and regain, to some extent, her senses. It is noteworthy that the Town Court of Kajaani acquitted Johan but still reprimanded him because they considered that it would have been more suitable for available 'older men and priests' to have been called upon for this purpose. In fact, the town mayor and the castle commandant had already used this method on Brita some days earlier, the first time in order to return her to her senses and the second time upon the request of her husband.[56] A similar 'cure that had good effect' was proposed by the provincial governor in Gävle in central Sweden in 1698. The cure consisted of forcing those who were 'raging and beset' (Swe. *rasande och besatte*) to recite the Lord's prayer and the Psalm 51, asking forgiveness for sins, on pain of whipping. Whipping was allowed until the person appeared docile and compliant; the king permitted the use of this treatment.[57] These references show that prayer was deemed so important that even physical discipline was allowed and encouraged. Moreover, they suggest that whipping the mad, in particular those suffering from raving

55 See also Houston, *Madness and Society*, 293–297, 311–315; Miettinen, 'Constructing "Mad" Religious Experiences.'

56 Case described in Manninen, 'Ylioppilas parantajana' and, briefly, in Pietikäinen, *Hulluuden historia*, 52–53.

57 Sandholm, *Kyrkan och hospitalshjonen*, 245.

madness, 'into their senses' was an old custom that was appropriate at least when carried out by state office holders.

The significance of prayer also comes across vividly in the notes of Nils Gissler, a doctor who treated both his own afflictions as well as some 'mad' patients in the 1750s and 1760s. His treatments included the use of chemical and herbal substances, bloodletting, and diverse spiritual treatments. He found 'self-help' from reading the New Testament and various other biblical passages and devotional literature. Gissler associated most of the conditions and symptoms he treated with the Devil, although he considered that it was difficult to distinguish between those deriving from 'natural' illness and those supported by devilish forces. First and foremost, he recommended full confession of sins and 'holding the patient on prayer and to God's word.' The treatments included repeatedly reading aloud prayers, for example, from the Book of Psalms or from Johan Arndt's prayerbook. Some patients also required examining and being taught the basic tenets of Lutheran faith. In a few cases, the similar kind of whipping and forced reciting of prayers, as practised by the student above, was deemed necessary. For example, Gissler treated a retired boatswain, who had been kept in chains due to his raving madness for three years, by reading prayers from Arndt's book aloud and giving him medicine several times a day but lashing him when he was wild and did not comply. This treatment lasted for three weeks, and ultimately, the man was able to read the prayer book and Luther's Small Catechism by himself.[58]

Gissler cooperated with the local clergy who also delivered spiritual therapies. Crucial for healing, Giessler considered both the religious counsel he and the clergy provided as well as the enthusiastic, personal prayer uttered by the 'mad' and afflicted themselves essential. Gissler's activities are good examples of how doctors practised spiritual forms of healing alongside other treatments, just as the clergy could provide other medications.[59]

All these religious practices were encouraged and in line with Protestant ideas. However, there are references to various spiritual activities aimed at healing that express religious pluralism in the officially religiously uniform Lutheran Swedish Realm. Most importantly, folk healers practised healing or curative magic that was often accompanied by Christian prayers, blessings, charms, symbols, and objects. These healing rituals also entailed religious

58 Gissler, *Några minnets qwarlefwor*: the boatswain's case is at 45–46.

59 Gissler, *Några minnets qwarlefwor*, passim. For similar types of spiritual therapies provided by Richard Napier, a physician in early modern England, see MacDonald, *Mystical Bedlam*, esp. 220–223.

gestures, such as making the sign of the cross. Healing magic was practised widely throughout the period in question, and also used for healing the 'mad.'[60]

Moreover, even though many Catholic traditions, such as pilgrimages and worship of saints, had been officially rejected in post-Reformation Sweden, these healing practices continued. Offerings made for healing, for example to certain churches that were considered particularly efficient in this respect, remained throughout the early modern period.[61] Offerings were made to alleviate all kinds of ailments. For example, in 1687 fines and ecclesiastical punishments were imposed on two women because they had made offerings on a holy day at the church altar, one for her daughter who was suffering from falling sickness and the other for her daughter suffering from an eye condition. The women explained that they had 'sought help in Jesus' name' and simply acted following an old practice, doing what many other locals had done and had found remedy for their ailments.[62] Likewise, the Christian tradition and rite of exorcism continued, although it was an unorthodox and illicit practice. As mentioned, it was widely accepted that the Devil could inflict, cause, or fool someone into madness (or other illnesses), and even, most drastically, possess people. However, the practice of exorcism appears to have been rare.[63]

Although this chapter has mostly been about healing that incorporated religious features, it must be emphasised that they were only one part of all the activities that the 'ill,' including the mad, practised in order to alleviate

60 Toivo, *Faith and Magic*, esp. 42–50; Van Gent, *Magic, Body, and the Self*, esp. 127–149; Zachrisson, *Mellan fromhet och vidskepelse*. For example, a mother sought help from a folk healer for her disturbed daughter, but it only worsened her condition. Gissler, *Några minnets qwarlefwor*, 36. On women involved in magical healing and popular medicine in early modern Europe, see Whaley, *Women and the Practice*, 174–195.

61 About the continuing offering practices, and offering churches, in early modern Sweden, see Toivo, *Faith and Magic*, esp. 50–60; Weikert, *I sjukdom och nöd*; Zachrisson, 'Images,' 112–115. See also Zachrisson, 'The Saint' and Zachrisson, 'Visiting Holy Wells.' Objects and money were donated both for healing and for giving thanks for recovery or other fortune. E.g., a man suffering from 'weakness in the head' for over two years said to his friends that he would give the church some money if he got better. KA: RT Northern Ostrobothnia KO a 41: 1275–1289, Ii and Pudasjärvi, 8–13 March 1725.

62 KA: RT Ylä-Satakunta KO a 9: 348–349, Orivesi, 2 September 1687.

63 Some cases from early modern Sweden are presented in Eriksson, *Vägen till centralhospitalet*, 80–83 (two exorcisms of mad women in 1701 and 1714); Manninen, 'Ylioppilas parantajana' (the presented student's case from 1730 also included phrases about driving the devil out); and Matikainen, 'Kurkijoen manaajapappi' (rumours and claims of various exorcism activities of a priest in the 1640s). On possessed people in later Finnish folklore, see, e.g., Klemettinen, *Mellastavat pirut*, 127–130.

or recover from their condition. Different practices were in use side by side, usually not competing with but complementing each other. A good example of the plurality in healing, and about the interaction between 'spiritual' and other cures, comes from southwestern Sweden. In 1707, Gunla, a soldier's wife in her forties, was frequently visited by the local clergy, including the pastor and the chaplain, who 'through the comfort of God's Word tried to free her from' her melancholia. In addition, a barber-surgeon had practised bloodletting to ease her condition. Gunla had also sought 'peace and relief for her great anguish' by visiting and talking with her sister and brother-in-law. During Gunla's visit there, in another locality, the local chaplain was invited over to 'console her with God's Word' in the home of Gunla's sister and brother-in-law. Likewise, Gunla had been prayed for in the local church.[64]

Conclusion

The chapter has shown that in early modern Sweden, faith, religious practice, and 'spiritual physic' were considered vital not only for upholding health but also for recovering from ill-health, including illnesses and conditions that were connected to madness. Faith and religious rituals had manifold functions in 'healthcare.' They maintained and improved well-being, helped the ill to recover through God's mercy, and aided them in battling against ailments caused by demonic forces. Alongside their perceived health benefits, faith and religious practices also offered the patient solace and spiritual consolation. These views were in line with the scholarly medicine and the mainstream Lutheran thinking of the period.

The scarcity and lack of access to scholarly medicine left plenty of room for ordinary people to turn to various strategies. As the vast majority of the mentally disturbed resided outside hospitals, asylums, or other poor relief institutions, healing was carried out primarily at homes, villages, and churches. Based on the sources, healing practices that entailed religious rituals and spiritual elements were not uncommon among the peasantry in early modern Sweden. The practices in healing the 'insane' abundantly manifest both the medical pluralism and the significance of religion and faith in early modern Sweden. Even if other healing activities, like

64 Lower court records of Sundal, 4 September 1707 in Sjödahl and Edestam, *Ur Sundals härads domböcker*, 84. About combining religious and humoral healing methods in sixteenth-century Sweden, see Gabriela Bjarne Larsson's chapter in this volume.

bloodletting or medications, were deployed, faith and religious practice were considered crucial; after all, God had the ultimate power over health and recovery.

Although scientific notions related to medicine, healing and the aetiology of illnesses underwent some changes during the long period of over a century (c. 1600s–1730s), the conceptions and practices in the local communities are nevertheless characterised by continuities. Beliefs in demonic forces causing madness and mental disturbances persisted. Most importantly, prayer and other spiritual healing activities remained commonplace throughout the period.

These healing practices at the local level are another example of lived religion, that is, how religion was carried out and performed in everyday life in early modern Sweden. Prayer, hymn singing, and other religious rituals were in used in finding relief and alleviation for mental illnesses and disturbances. Pastoral counselling and intermediation was also considered important. Visits to and by the clergy were expected and not uncommon. Tending to the ill and afflicted, by way of pastoral visitations and consolation and through organising communal prayers at church, was an important task performed by the local clergy. These were approved orthodox Lutheran practices that were performed to cure and treat the ill community members; their use not only demonstrates the significance of orthodoxy in itself during this period but also strengthened and reconstructed the ideal and appropriate practice of faith and religion.

Alongside these appropriate spiritual healing practices, which were encouraged in medical and ecclesiastical treatises, spiritual cures that the authorities considered Catholic, superstitious, or magic were also in use. We can assume that there were regional and social differences in the vast Realm, both regarding access to clergy and religious spaces and, for example, in the customary and familiar healing practices of localities and areas. Moreover, most of the tracked cases involve landed and/or elderly locals who appear to have had long-lasting ties in the congregation in which they received the accepted Christian and Lutheran religious remedies. Perhaps their established status gave them more access to clergymen and services compared to, for example, landless servants, labourers, and newcomers. On the other hand, it is similarly possible that it was primarily the most pious who sought spiritual means of healing for their and their family members' ailments.

Furthermore, the cases suggest that there was some selectivity as to which types of madness required or deserved more clerical attention and more fervent personal religious practice. The local clergy appear to have been actively involved especially in cases of those whose madness was attributed to devilish forces and in cases of melancholia. Moreover, especially those suffering from raving madness were prescribed, and forced to perform, repeated recitations of prayers. It is possible that these conditions were closely associated with spiritual and supernatural causes and forces in the thinking of the era. This suggests that the interpreted instigator or cause of the illness influenced which method of healing was selected, as well as the extent of pastoral involvement and spiritual healing necessary. In the case of melancholia, the clergy were experts to tend the symptoms of this ailment. This condition might also include supernatural forces as well as unfavourable spiritual thinking which needed intervention. Nevertheless, there were many who suffered from other, undetermined mental weaknesses, who were also receiving clerical consolation, were prayed for and who practised religion in order to heal.

As we have seen, religion had an integral part in healthcare in early modern Swedish society. The idea of faith healing also implied communal significance because it offered a means by which the local communities could participate in the healing process. Like the local clergy, families, friends, and parishioners continued to have an intermediary role because they could engage in healing, especially via praying for the ill at church and elsewhere.

Bibliography

Archival sources

The Hagströmer Medico-Historical Library, Karolinska Institutet, Stockholm
KIB MS 69:1. Nils Gissler. *Några minnets qwarlefwor af det som genom Guds nådiga skickelse tildragit sig under min långwariga siuklighet ifrån 1751 til närwarande tid.*
Provincial Archives of Uppsala (Landsarkivet i Uppsala, ULA)
Kopparberg läns häradsrätts arkiv.
Uppsala länsstyrelsens arkiv.
Örebro länsstyrelsens arkiv.
Riksarkivet, National Archives of Sweden (RA)
Svea Hovrätt Advokatfiskalens arkiv: Collections of *Renoverade domböcker* (SHA).
National Archives of Finland (Kansallisarkisto, KA)
Collections of *Renoverade domböcker* (RT)

Printed works

Balduin, Friedrich. *Samwetz plåster emoot allahanda samwetz-quaal in genere et in specie: Doch särdeles them, som twijfla om sina ewigha saligheet, så ock them som leedas wid at leffua, och wela sigh sielffua förgöra*. Translated into Swedish by Ericus Matthiae. Wästerås, 1638 [1628]. Digitised at: https://digital.ub.umu.se/node/178918/.

Church Law of 1686. In Samfundet Pro fide et christianismo (utg.). *1686 års kyrkolag med inledning av Gabriel Thulin*. Stockholm: Svenska kyrkans diakonistyrelse, 1936. Also transcribed and digitised at: http://www.mlang.name/arkisto/kyrkiolag-1686.html.

Colerus, Johannes. *Oeconomia, Thet är Hushåldz Underwijsning För 40 Åhr sedan Förswänskat Och i många Rum uthaf andra authoribus amplificerat och förbättrat af Isaaco Erici, Pastore Stenbyense i Östergötland*. Translated into Swedish by Isaacus Erici. Stockholm, 1683 [1591].

De Britaine, William. *Klokhets och skyldighets reglor eller Mennisklig försichtighet och konst, hwarigenom en menniskios lycka kan befordras*. Stockholm, 1743 [orig. *On Human Prudence, or the Way by which a Man may raise himself to Fortune and Grandeur*, 1693]. Translated into Swedish and printed since 1725. Digitised at: https://digital.ub.umu.se/resolve?urn=urn:17a_000014.

Gyllenius, Petrus M. *Diarium Gyllenianum eller Petrus Magni Gyllenii Dagbok 1622–1667*, edited by R. Hausen. Utg. Finska Statsarkivet genom Reinh. Hausen. Helsinki, 1882 [1622–1667].

Handbok 1693. *Handbok, ther uti är författat, huruledes gudztiensten, med christelige ceremonier och kyrkcioseder, uti wåra swenska församlingar skal blifwa hållen och förhandlad: förbättrad och förmehrad i Stockholm åhr 1599, öfversedd åhr 1608, och nymera efter nyja kyrckio-ordningen inrättad åhr 1693*. Stockholm: J. R. Horrn, 1735.

Hemmingsen, Niels. *Antidotum. Thet Är: En Saligh Läkedom Och Tröst, Emoot Then Farligha Och Förgifftigha Siälennes Siukdom, Som Är Misströst, Eller Förtwifan Om Gudz Nådhe Och Syndernas Förlåtelse*. Stockholm, 1608.

Hjärne, Urban. *Een uthförlig Berättelse om the nyys opfundne Suurbrunnar widh Medewij uthi Östergöthland, huru the bäst skole brukas, ... therjämpte några nödwändige frågor och ytterst några förledne åhrs curer opteknade*. Stockholm, 1680. Digitised at: http://www.alvin-portal.org/alvin/view.jsf?pid=alvin-record%3A104718&dswid=-2667.

Lindh, Carl. *Huusz-apoteek och läkie-book, hwar uthi allehanda hälsosamma rådh och på många meniskior offta proberade läkedommar, ... och på hwad sätt de kunna botas*. Wijsingzborg, 1675.

Olai, Benedictus. *Een Nyttigh Läkere Book. Faksimiledition, med inledning av O. T. Hult*. Edited by John Kroon. Malmö: Malmö Ljustrycksanstalt, 1938 [1578].

Sjödahl, Elsa, and Anders Edestam, eds. *Ur Sundals härads domböcker 1700–1730*. Färjelanda: Dalslands fornminnes- och hembygdsförbund, 1995.

Sparman [Palmkron], Andreas. *Sundhetzens speghel, uthi hwilken man beskodhar Sundhetzens Natur, förnämste Orsakerne til alla Siukdomar, om Sundheten förstöra plåga; såsom ock the Medels rätta bruk*. Stockholm, 1686 [1642].

Tranaeus, Johan Gottskalck. *Medewij suurbrunnars märckwärdige curer, på desze tre sista åhren ....* Stockholm, 1690.

Triewald, Mårten. 'Rön angående Camphers stora ock underbara värkan i Mania eller hos Månads rasande Människor.' *Kungl. (Svenska) Vetenskapsakademiens Handlingar* (1744): 53–57.

Literature

Annola, Johanna, and Riikka Miettinen. 'Piety and Prayers: Religion in the Lives of the Indoor Poor in Finland, 1600s–1960s.' In *Lutheranism and Social Responsibility*, edited by Nina Javette Koefoed and Andrew Newby, 129–152. Refo500 Academic Studies 82. Göttingen: Vandenhoeck & Ruprecht, 2022.

Classen, Albrecht, ed. *Mental Health, Spirituality, and Religion in the Middle Ages and Early Modern Age*. Fundamentals of Medieval and Early Modern Culture 15. Berlin and Boston: De Gruyter, 2014.

Cunningham, Andrew, and Ole Peter Grell, eds. *Medicine and Religion in Enlightenment Europe*. Aldershot: Ashgate, 2007.

Cunningham, Andrew, and Ole Peter Grell, eds. *'Religio Medici': Medicine and Religion in Seventeenth-Century England*. Aldershot: Scolar Press, 1996.

De Waardt, Hans. 'Chasing Demons and Curing Mortals: The Medical Practice of Clerics in the Netherlands.' In *The Task of Healing. Medicine, Religion and Gender in England and the Netherlands 1450–1800*, edited by Hilary Marland and Margaret Pelling, 171–203. Rotterdam: Erasmus Publishing, 1996.

Duffin, Jacalyn. *Medical Miracles. Doctors, Saints and Healing in the Modern World*. Oxford: Oxford University Press, 2008.

Eilola, Jari. 'Defining and Treating Madness in Local Communities Early Modern Finland.' In *Encountering Crises of the Mind. Madness, Culture and Society, 1200s–1900s*, edited by Tuomas Laine-Frigren, Jari Eilola, and Markku Hokkanen, 69–87. Leiden: Brill, 2019.

Eriksson, Bengt Erik. *Vägen till centralhospitalet. Två studier om den anstaltsbundna sinnessjukvårdens förhistoria i Sverige*. Gothenburg: Daidalos, 1989.

Gentilcore, David. *Healers and Healing in Early Modern Italy* Manchester: Manchester University Press, 1998.

Grell, Ole Peter. 'Caspar Bartholin and the Education of the Pious Physician.' In *Medicine and the Reformation*, edited by Ole Peter Grell and Andrew Cunningham, 78–100. London: Routledge, 1993.

Grell, Ole Peter, and Andrew Cunningham, eds. *Medicine and the Reformation*. London: Routledge, 1993.

Harley, David. 'Spiritual Physic, Providence, and English Medicine, 1560–1640.' In *Medicine and the Reformation*, edited by Ole Peter Grell and Andrew Cunningham, 101–117. London: Routledge, 1993.

Hayward, Rhodri. 'Psychiatry and Religion.' In *The Routledge History of Madness and Mental Health*, edited by Greg Eghigian, 137–152. London: Routledge, 2017.

Hodgkin, Katherine. *Madness in Seventeenth-Century Autobiography*. Basingstoke: Palgrave Macmillan, 2007.

Houston, R. A. *Madness and Society in Eighteenth-Century Scotland*. Oxford: Oxford University Press, 2000.

Ingram, Allan. 'Deciphering Difference: A Study in Medical Literacy.' In *Melancholy Experience in Literature of the Long Eighteenth Century. Before Depression, 1660–1800*, edited by Allan Ingram, Stuart Sim, Clark Lawlor, Richard Terry, John Baker, and Leigh Wetherall-Dickson, 170–202. Basingstoke: Palgrave Macmillan, 2011.

Jimenez, Mary Ann. *Changing Faces of Madness: Early American Attitudes and Treatment of the Insane*. Hanover: University Press of New England for Brandeis University Press, 1987.

Joutsivuo, Timo. 'Ruumiin vai sielun hoitoa? Kristinusko, sairaus ja lääketiede.' In *Terveyden lähteillä. Länsimaisten terveyskäsitysten kulttuurihistoriaa*, edited by Timo Joutsivuo and Heikki Mikkeli, 59–83. Helsinki: The Finnish Literature Society, 1998.

Kassell, Lauren, and Robert Ralley. 'Prayer and Physic in Seventeenth-Century England.' *Early Science and Medicine* 26, nos. 5–6 (2021): 480–508.

Katajala-Peltomaa, Sari. *Demonic Possession and Lived Religion in Later Medieval Europe*. Oxford: Oxford University Press, 2020.

Katajala-Peltomaa, Sari, and Raisa Maria Toivo. 'Introduction: Religion as Historical Experience.' In *Histories of Experience in the World of Religion*, edited by Sari Katajala-Peltomaa and Raisa Maria Toivo, 1–35. Palgrave Studies in the History of Experience. London: Palgrave Macmillan, 2022.

Katajala-Peltomaa, Sari, and Raisa Maria Toivo. 'Religion as Experience.' In *Lived Religion and the Long Reformation in Northern Europe c. 1300–1700*, edited by Sari Katajala-Peltomaa and Raisa Maria Toivo, 1–18. Leiden: Brill, 2017.

Klemettinen, Pasi. *Mellastavat pirut. Tutkimus kansanomaisista paholais- ja noituuskäsityksistä Karjalan kannaksen ja Laatokan Karjalan tarinaperinteessä*. Helsinki: The Finnish Literature Society, 1997.

Lederer, David. *Madness, Religion and the State in Early Modern Europe: A Bavarian Beacon*. Cambridge: Cambridge University Press, 2006.

Lederer, David. 'Psychiatry in the Sixteenth Century? Spiritual Physic in Early Modern Europe.' In *Historia de la Psiquiatría en Europa: Temas y tendencias*, edited by F. Fuentenebro de Diego, R. Huertas Garcia-Alejo, and C. Valiente Ots, 79–86. Madrid: Frenia, 2003.

Lindemann, Mary. *Medicine and Society in Early Modern Europe*. 2nd ed. Cambridge: Cambridge University Press, 2010.

MacDonald, Michael. *Mystical Bedlam: Madness, Anxiety, and Healing in Seventeenth-Century England*. Cambridge: Cambridge University Press, 1981.

MacDonald, Michael. 'Religion, Social Change, and Psychological Healing in England, 1600–1800.' *Studies in Church History* 19, 'The Church and Healing' (1982): 101–125.

Manninen, Ohto. 'Ylioppilas parantajana eli houruinhoitoa 1700-luvulla.' *Hippokrates* 3 (1986), 88–97.

Matikainen, Olli. 'Kurkijoen manaajapappi.' In *Manaajista maalaisaateliin. Tulkintoja toisesta historian, antropologian ja maantieteen välimaastosta*, edited by Kimmo Katajala, 163–180. Helsinki: The Finnish Literature Society, 1995.

Mellyn, Elizabeth W. 'Healers and Healing in the Early Modern Health Care Market.' In *The Routledge History of Madness and Mental Health*, edited by Greg Eghigian, 83–100. London: Routledge, 2017.

Mellyn, Elizabeth W. *Mad Tuscans and Their Families: A History of Mental Disorder in Early Modern Italy*. Philadelphia: University of Pennsylvania Press, 2014.

Miettinen, Riikka. 'Constructing "Mad" Religious Experiences in Early Modern Sweden.' In *Histories of Experience in the World of Religion*, edited by Sari Katajala-Peltomaa and Raisa Maria Toivo, 163–194. Palgrave Studies in the History of Experience. London: Palgrave Macmillan, 2022.

Miettinen, Riikka. *Suicide, Law, and Community in Early Modern Sweden*. Basingstoke: Palgrave Macmillan, 2019.

Mortimer, Ian. *The Dying and the Doctors: The Medical Revolution in Seventeenth-Century England*. Woodbridge: Royal Historical Society Publications, 2009.

Newton, Hannah. *Misery to Mirth: Recovery from Illness in Early Modern England*. Oxford: Oxford University Press, 2018.

Peschier, Diana. *Lost Souls: Women, Religion and Mental Illness in the Victorian Asylum*. London: Bloomsbury Publishing, 2019.

Pietikäinen, Petteri. *Hulluuden historia*. Helsinki: Gaudeamus, 2013. Translated into English as *Madness: A History*. London: Routledge, 2015.

Ross, Tricia Marie. *Care of Bodies, Cure of Souls: Medicine and Religion in Early Modern Germany*. PhD diss., Duke University, 2017. Retrieved from https://hdl.handle.net/10161/14494.

Sandholm, Åke. *Kyrkan och hospitalshjonen. En undersökning rörande omsorgen om de sjuka och fattiga i välfärdsanstalterna i Finland*. Finska Kyrkohistoriska Samfundets handlingar 88. Helsinki: Finska Kyrkohistoriska Samfundets, 1973.

Schmidt, Jeremy. *Melancholy and the Care of the Soul: Religion, Moral Philosophy and Madness in Early Modern England*. The History of Medicine in Context. Aldershot: Ashgate, 2007.

Stolberg, Michael. *Experiencing Illness and the Sick Body in Early Modern Europe*. Basingstoke: Palgrave Macmillan, 2011.

Sundmark, Stina Fallberg. *Sjukbesök och dödsberedelse: sockenbudet i svensk medeltida och reformatorisk tradition*. Bibliotheca theologiae practicae 84. Skellefteå: Artos, 2008.

Svenska Akademiens Ordbok (*SAOB*). Swedish Academy Dictionary, online: https://www.saob.se/.

Thomas, Keith. *Religion and the Decline of Magic: Studies in Popular Beliefs in Sixteenth- and Seventeenth-Century England*. London: Penguin, 1971.

Toivo, Raisa Maria. *Faith and Magic in Early Modern Finland*. Basingstoke: Palgrave Macmillan, 2016.

Van Gent, Jacqueline. *Magic, Body, and the Self in Eighteenth-Century Sweden*. Leiden: Brill, 2009.

Wear, Andrew. 'Puritan Perceptions of Illness in Seventeenth Century England.' In *Patients and Practitioners: Lay Perceptions of Medicine in Pre-industrial Society*, edited by Roy Porter, 55–101. Cambridge: Cambridge University Press, 1985.

Wear, Anthony. 'Religious Beliefs and Medicine in Early Modern England.' In *The Task of Healing. Medicine, Religion and Gender in England and the Netherlands 1450–1800*, edited by Hilary Marland and Margaret Pelling, 145–169. Rotterdam: Erasmus, 1996.

Weatherhead, Lesley. *Psychology, Religion and Healing*. London: Hodder & Stoughton, 1959.

Weikert, Monica. *I sjukdom och nöd. Offerkyrkoseden i Sverige från 1600-tal till 1800-tal*. Gothenburg: Göteborgs universitet, 2004.

Whaley, Leigh. *Women and the Practice of Medical Care in Early Modern Europe, 1400–1800*. Basingstoke: Palgrave Macmillan, 2011.

Zachrisson, Terese. 'Images, "Superstition," and Popular Piety in Post-Reformation Sweden.' *Mirator* 19, no. 1 (2018): 108–118.

Zachrisson, Terese. *Mellan fromhet och vidskepelse: Materialitet och religiositet i det efterreformatoriska Sverige*. Gothenburg: University of Gothenburg, Faculty of Arts, Department of Historical Studies, 2017.

Zachrisson, Terese. 'The Saint in the Woods: Semi-Domestic Shrines in Rural Sweden, c. 1500–1800.' *Religions* 10, no. 6 (2019): 386. https://doi.org/10.3390/rel10060386.
Zachrisson, Terese. 'Visiting Holy Wells in Seventeenth-Century Sweden: The Case of St. Ingemo's Well in Dala.' In *Sacred Waters: A Cross-Cultural Compendium of Hallowed Springs and Holy Wells*, edited by Celeste Ray, 318–327. London: Routledge, 2020.

About the Author

Riikka Miettinen works as a Senior Research Fellow at the Centre of Excellence in the History of Experiences based at Tampere University, Finland. Her current research projects deal with the history of madness, lived religion, and disability in early modern Sweden and Finland.

7. Not Quacks but Close: Reappraising the Role of Physicians on the Eighteenth-Century Medical Market

Hjalmar Fors

Abstract

This chapter reassesses the relationship between physicians and the eighteenth-century Swedish state. It argues that physicians' connection to the state was rather tenuous throughout the period, and that they were neither considered nor treated as an important part of the cameralist machine of governance. This is a position which runs contrary to earlier historiography, which has tended to portray eighteenth-century physicians as forerunners to nineteenth- and twentieth-century branches of the state that are concerned with social medicine, hygiene, and general improvement of the health of the population. By giving examples of how physicians operated in different roles on the Swedish medical market and in relation to the state, the chapter points to the sprawling complexity of early modern health practices.

Keywords: eighteenth-century medicine, Enlightenment, medical market, social medicine

Introduction

Physicians often tend to be seen as holding the top position in the hierarchy of health practitioners. In prior research, they often come across as aloof, high-status figures, who in the eighteenth-century paired up with the state to regulate, oversee, and improve the activities of all other health practitioners.[1] This chapter argues that Swedish physicians' connection to

1 Classical overviews which to a large degree still shape more recent narratives are Hjelt, *Svenska och finska*, vols. 1–3; Ahlberg, *Den Svenska farmaciens*; Kock, ed., *Medicinalväsendet i*

Eyice, M. and C. Forss (eds.), *Health and Society in Early Modern Sweden*.
Taylor & Francis Group 2024
DOI 10.5117/9789463724296_CH07

the state remained tenuous throughout the eighteenth century. I contend that physicians were not particularly important to the state, *except as* one of many groups of actors on a medical market.[2] They were, to put it bluntly, neither considered nor treated as an important part of the machine of governance. That is not to say that they were completely unimportant, but neither were hatters, cobblers, or indeed barber-surgeons or midwives inconsequential. This, of course, is a position that runs contrary to earlier historiography, which has tended to portray eighteenth-century physicians, and in particular their main organisation the Collegium Medicum, as forerunners to nineteenth- and twentieth-century branches of the state that are concerned with social medicine, hygiene, and general improvement of the health of the population. By giving examples of how physicians negotiated with other groups and operated in different roles on the Swedish medical market and in relation to the state, this chapter instead points to the sprawling complexity and open-ended nature of early modern health practices. To create a more complex, and hopefully also more truthful, description of the role of physicians in eighteenth-century Swedish society, I take as my point of departure two propositions, which underlie the argument of the present chapter.

My first proposition is that we should leave aside the notion of the high status of physicians and study the physicians' attempts to distinguish themselves from other practitioners as a multifaceted and fluctuating process. The high status of physicians was indeed established by the end of the eighteenth century – but the process leading to this elevated position was neither linear nor obvious.[3] Thus, the chapter begins by situating the Collegium Medicum in relation to the Swedish state and other groups of knowledge-holders that were connected to the Swedish state apparatus. The main question here is: How did physicians, in their social role and their reforming efforts, compare to those state officials who wielded much more influence, and were decidedly nearer to the center of state power?

My second proposition is that earlier literature about the emergence of physicians' organisations and institutions is skewed, due to its overly

Sverige; Lindroth, *Svensk Lärdomshistoria: Frihetstiden*. Some more recent works which partially problematise the inherited view without wholly rejecting it are Ling, *Kärringmedicin*; Gustafsson, *Läkaren, döden*; Widenberg, *Den stora kreatursdöden*.

2 For the concept *medical market* as applied to eighteenth-century Sweden, and the physicians' difficulties to make inroads as actors in midwifery, see Paulsson Holmberg, *Onaturlig födelse*, 15–20, 88–92.

3 The chapter develops several themes explored in a previous work, which focused on the seventeenth century. See Fors, 'Medicine.'

narrow focus on the role of physicians as regulators and inspectors of other practitioners. This skewed historiography naturally elevates the status and role of physicians in relation to other health practitioners. Deliberately or inadvertently, such narratives tend to portray physicians as aloof and truth-seeking arbiters of medical knowledge. I will not assume, a priori, that physicians' agendas, whether personal or as a corporation, are radically different from those of any other groups of medical practitioners. Aiming for symmetry of description I will discuss some examples in which physicians' medical and commercial practices infringed on the fields of other practitioners, or even bordered on the illicit.[4] In this way, the chapter arrives at a particular perspective; namely, that physicians may not have enjoyed such high status in eighteenth-century Sweden after all, and may, in practice, have been difficult to distinguish from other groups of health practitioners (others being travelling quacks, midwives, barber-surgeons, dentists, apothecaries, bathers, and so on). From this line of reasoning follows the notion that historiography has made too much of physicians' construction of professional identity and loyalty to their professional group, and that historians should pay more attention to physicians' individual economic activities and devotion and loyalty to family and patronage networks.[5]

Physicians wooing the state

Sweden was much diminished by war, famine, and plague during the decades around 1700, leaving the realm a shadow of its former seventeenth-century martial glory. However, Stockholm remained an important centre of medical activity, and knowledge.[6] Thus, midwives from Finland regularly travelled to Stockholm to learn their art and take their certification exam.[7] Similarly,

4 I.e., the chapter proceeds theoretically from the strong programme of the sociology of knowledge as formulated by Bloor, *Knowledge and Social Imagery*. See also Fors, *Limits*, 7–11.

5 There is a rather large body of recent work which has reassessed patronage and clientism in eighteenth-century Sweden. For discussions of scientific and medical practitioners, see Hodacs and Nyberg, *Naturalhistoria*, esp. 109–119; Fors 'Matematiker mot linneaner,' 25–53; Orrje, *Mechanicus*, 158–198; Windahl Pontén, *Kiär hustru*, esp. 120–136.

6 With its c. 70,000 inhabitants at the middle of the eighteenth century, it was also a significant Baltic city, and Sweden's largest by far. Gothenburg, for example, held no more than c. 10,000 inhabitants. Fritz, 'Göteborg,' 12.

7 Vainio-Korhonen, *De frimodiga*, 12, 28–32, 37, 40–42, 47, 50, 67–114.

Stockholm held the largest concentration of physicians, barber-surgeons, and apothecaries in the realm. The city was also, from 1663, the seat of the Swedish Collegium Medicum, which had evolved from being – more or less – a corporation of Stockholm physicians with a Royal Charter (in the seventeenth century) into something which, at least on the surface, was in the eighteenth century more akin to a state body, governing and overseeing all medical practitioners of the realm.[8]

Seventeenth-century Sweden's community of physicians was small, and largely confined to Stockholm, as well as to university faculties in Uppsala, Lund, Åbo (Fin. Turku) and Greifswald. Thus, there was little opportunity for this community to move beyond or expand upon its primary role as health advisors to an elite clientele. During the eighteenth century, there was a marked expansion of their number. Already in the previous century, some larger towns had hired town physicians, who were expected to gain the main part of their income from private practice but were given a complementary salary paid by local authorities. The office of province physician had been mentioned already in a Royal Ordnance of 1688; the establishment of the position was an initiative taken to improve the healthcare situation in the countryside. But the system was slow to be enacted. In 1723, only twelve existed nationwide. Province physicians still had no formal directives, and most of them were town physicians who were assigned an additional title and task, but still employed and paid by the towns in which they resided. Their numbers increased from then on, and eventually there was a general overhaul of the province physician system (1773). Forty districts (of which eight were in Finland) were created. Just as in the previous century, province physicians were expected to earn the larger part of their income through their private practice. But as patients often were lacking, or as the case would be, preferred to seek the services of other health practitioners, these physicians often supplemented their income with complementary activities such as teaching in schools.[9] But there is no denying that the profession and its status was in ascendancy during the eighteenth century. In the 1780s, there were about 140 physicians in the Swedish realm, and towards the end of

8 Fors, 'Medicine.' The sticking point was that *Collegium Medicum* was subordinated to and inspected by the county governor (Swe. *Överståthållaren*) of Stockholm. Hjelt, *Svenska och Finska*, 1:15.

9 See Lindroth, *Svensk Lärdomshistoria: Frihetstiden*, 420–21; Hjelt, *Svenska och finska*, 1:60–61, 496–511; Hjelt, *Svenska och finska*, 2:11–20, 23–25, 135. Province physicians were also connected to the state through forensic medicine (*medicina legalis*) after it became part of their duties to provide medical advice to the legal authorities. See also Gustafsson, *Läkaren, döden*, 19–20.

the century, Stockholm (pop. c. 73,000) had amassed sixty physicians – a considerable number.[10]

When it was founded in the mid-seventeenth century, the Collegium Medicum had been more or less a guild-like corporation that organised the physicians of Stockholm. Its founding charter gave the physicians the exclusive privilege to practise internal medicine in the city. In addition, they were given the right to inspect all other groups of medical practitioners who were suspected of practising internal medicine or treating external symptoms that were likely to have internal causes.[11] However, soon apothecaries and barber-surgeons mounted successful campaigns to circumscribe the influence of the physicians, and physicians' attempts to gain control over their professions. It was only with the Royal Ordnance of 1698 that a truce between these rivaling factions was finally called. The Collegium was now acknowledged to be an organisation of national scope, but the Ordnance also contained concessions to apothecaries and barber-surgeons. Both groups were given extensive privileges to provide healthcare of various types. The physicians' exclusive privilege to practise internal medicine was only to be upheld when they were available or close by, and it seems that the Ordinance was deliberately vague on what was meant with the availability of physicians. Thus, apothecaries were permitted to serve the public both with advice and in practice, when no physician was available, and barber-surgeons were permitted to work as physicians in such places where no physicians with a medical degree could be found.[12]

In the following decades, the physicians of the Collegium made several attempts to transform their organisation into a proper branch of government in the form of a Bureau, (Swe. *Kollegium*) of the central state apparatus. They deemed this to be important, as it would also give them the title of *assessors*, and thus a formal rank in the Swedish state hierarchy. Further aims were to have an executive, rather than merely advisory, function, and to receive reimbursement from the state for their work as well as funds to pay a scribe or clerk to record their minutes. They also wanted to be provided with an office or meeting room and the firewood to keep it warm. The formal title of assessor was granted in 1719, but as late as the 1730s, the state refused outright to provide the Collegium with new offices and a meeting room. This forced the physicians to meet in their private homes, as they generally

10 Lindroth, *Svensk Lärdomshistoria: Frihetstiden* 421; Hjelt, *Svenska och finska*, 2:3–11.

11 Riksregistraturet 1663 part 2, fol. 34, published in Hjelt, *Svenska och finska*, 1:10–14. See also ibid., 8–9, 326–327.

12 Ahlberg, *Svenska farmaciens*, 55, 87; Hjelt, *Svenska och finska*, 1:9–27.

had done in the seventeenth century. As I have discussed elsewhere, these early attempts to gain recognition and authority established only a tenuous connection to the state.[13] Traditional historiography, however, has tended to describe the members of Collegium Medicum of the seventeenth and eighteenth centuries as state officials, or as state officials in waiting.[14] This is not entirely incorrect, but it obscures important facts, some of which have already been touched upon. The most important of these facts is that the Collegium was primarily an advisory body without executive functions. For most intents and purposes, it was also a body of local – that is, Stockholm – influence which did not answer directly to the national authorities. Its immediate superior was the County Governor of Stockholm (Swe. *Överståthållaren*), whose responsibility included to oversee the city's guilds. This state of affairs – and in particular the Collegium's subordination to the County Governor of Stockholm – clearly implies that well into the eighteenth century, many saw the organisation as a guild for Stockholm physicians. In this context, the issue of salaries is illuminating, too. Unlike proper state officials – who, as a rule could expect salaried positions – the members of the Collegium worked for no payment until the 1760s, when they started to receive small salaries.[15] That the physicians were not the equals of other state officials was clearly spelled out in a Royal Letter declining a request for a salary increase in 1778:

> It has not escaped Our attention, that [...] your members, as they normally also are [medical] practitioners [...] are eligible for remunerations, [which] far more contribute to their income, than the salaries they enjoy from the Crown. Therefore, You should not have portrayed yourselves as the equals of Our, and the Crown's other officials, and you should not have applied for salaries on a par with theirs. Especially since the latter have no further permissible incomes from their office that they can use to assuage their needs, except their salaries.[16]

The Swedish state's message was clear. The physicians were first and foremost private practitioners, and as they received the larger part of their income on

13 Hjelt, *Svenska och finska*, 1:95; Fors, 'Medicine,' 488–492.

14 Hjelt, thus, does not seem to understand that the 1698 Ordnance was a product of compromise and negotiation. Hjelt, *Svenska och finska*, 1:27. See also ibid., 51, 72–73, and Sten Lindroth, *Svensk lärdomshistoria: Stormaktstiden*, 380–386, esp. 383.

15 Hjelt, *Svenska och finska*, 1:32, 99–101; Lindroth, *Svensk Lärdomshistoria: Frihetstiden*, 418.

16 Royal letter of 11 May 1778, quoted in Hjelt, *Svenska och finska*, 1:103 (my translation). All translations from Swedish to English are made by the author.

the medical market, they should presume neither the status nor the salary of other state officials. Indeed, the letter even describes the revenues of the physicians' private practice as permissible (Swe. *lofliga*) incomes received as a consequence of their state offices. It is a fine point which added insult to injury, as it further emphasised that the physicians were dependents who had received a privilege (i.e., Charter) to practise medicine from the state. Read in this way, the letter implied that the organisation of the physicians was a guild in need of state support. When such a harsh chastisement was delivered even in official Royal Letters, it is perhaps of little surprise that many of the Collegium's petitions and proposals were both ignored and regularly insulted by other, more influential officials and branches of government. As late as 1792, the Marshal of the Realm ranked the members of the Collegium as below those of the other Bureaus of the State and the fellows of Royal Academies.[17]

It was not just a matter of rank, but also of influence. Comparing the members of Collegium Medicum to the officials of one of the other state bureaus, the Bureau of Mines (Swe. *Bergskollegium*) for example, it seems clear that the officials of the latter held much more influence in the state, and in society. They, too, pursued collective and individual interests, but as properly salaried, high-status professionals. For instance, the officials of the Bureau of Mines were hardly competing with other actors in the mining business. As the state's representatives, the Bureau of Mines could command and direct over the state's subjects and draw on the full authority of the Crown to change laws and regulations when they deemed it proper to do so.[18] Although the physicians really wanted to have a similar position, appealing to the state and its representatives for it, and did all in their power to enact reforms, they did not succeed, at least not to any significant extent. The Collegium worked hard enough, but this work was, in a sense, conducted as a kind of mimicry of the work of the central bureaus of the state apparatus.

During the Swedish Age of Liberty (1719–1772), absolute monarchy was abolished and the center of political power moved instead to the Diet, or Riksdagen. Physicians were adept at orienting themselves in the emerging political, economic and epistemological landscape. Population management was a favorite trope in the *oeconomic* literature of the eighteenth century,

17 The issue of formal rank haunted the physicians throughout the seventeenth and eighteenth centuries and was not resolved until 1815. Hjelt, *Svenska och finska*, 1:72–85, 546–556. See also Cavallin, *I kungens*.

18 Fors, '"Away! Away to Falun!",' 557–563. Fors, *Limits*, 47–48, 101–109, 118.

and medicine – indeed, medical doctors – were deemed to have a role to play in political reform. In a discourse focusing on managing and developing natural resources, people were considered a key asset. To maximise the number of people within the realm, and to keep them in continuous, useful work, was considered a highly important, if not the most important, means to empower and strengthen the state.[19] A large, hardworking population was a key asset, and there were many ideas about how to achieve this goal through active policies of economic and societal reforms. The working people should consume as little as possible and salaries were to be held down, preferably lower than in other countries. On a more positive note, disease was to be held in check, too. Child mortality was identified as a main factor that prevented population growth and the means to prevent it were to be enacted.[20]

But the Collegium Medicum would not become the central organisation to direct reform efforts. A Royal Letter of 26 April 1737, decreed the creation of a special Commission for Health (Swe. *Sundhetskommissionen*). The commission was led by a Councillor of the Realm and senior politician, and its members included not only physicians, but also barber-surgeons and apothecaries. Until it was abolished in 1766, it would be the leading state actor in the field of medicine. It oversaw the province physicians, proposed reforms, and legislation, in particular with regard to countering epidemics and the spread of contagious disease, and was engaged in a great number of other tasks and projects.[21]

Thus, we can see that the Collegium was in fact pushed to the side as the leading government agency to oversee public health matters during a substantial part of the eighteenth century. This said, there was an overlap between the members of the Commission and the Collegium. Hence, the Stockholm physicians who dominated the Collegium did not really lose their connection with the state and the Diet. The Collegium also was prepared and ready to gain further official functions when opportunity arose. In a directive issued from the Diet to the Collegium in 1763, the body was instructed to transform itself into a node for gathering information about the health of the nation. Special attention was to be given to diseases and epidemics that reduced the population and diseases that killed the children of the common folk. Hospitals, orphanages, military barracks, and other similar institutions were to be inspected and information

19 Sandblad, *Världens nordligaste*, 3.

20 Lindroth, *Svensk Lärdomshistoria: Frihetstiden*, 414, 452.

21 Hjelt, *Svenska och finska*, 1:344–350. Hjelt, *Svenska och finska*, 2:12–13.

about these sites was to be gathered. The Collegium was also to supervise inoculation against smallpox and investigate why some occupations and parts of the country were more detrimental to health than others. All this information would be processed and forwarded to the Diet in the form of suggestions for reforms. In order to facilitate investigations, the Collegium was given full access to available national statistics (Swe. *Tabell- Wärket*), which had been proposed by the Swedish Royal Academy of Sciences and inaugurated in 1749.[22] The underlying rationale behind these changes was recognisably cameralist in nature. The Collegium was assigned to gather information through statistics, travelling, and reports. It was to summarise this information and forward it, together with suggestions for reforms, to the relevant decision makers.[23]

In this way, the physicians finally gained a measure of responsibility for public health. When the Commission for Health was abolished in 1766, the Collegium was instructed to take over both its archive and general field of responsibility. The Collegium was incorporated as a cog in the (imagined) machine of society. How big was this cog and did it perform any important tasks for the functioning of the machine? It is beyond the scope of this chapter to answer that question in depth. But it can be noted that although smallpox inoculation and other such similar measures may have had some public health impact, the toolbox of the eighteenth-century physician was rather limited. To put it in modern terms, the physicians of the period were mostly concerned with palliative care and dietetics on the individual level. With regards to the task to counter and treat epidemic and contagious disease, eighteenth-century medicine possessed few means to do this, apart from enforcing quarantine and distancing measures. Barber-surgeons and midwives, on the other hand, performed important daily societal functions such as binding wounds, setting bones, and delivering babies. These functions ensured the continuance of society, and propagation of the species. It remains to be ascertained to what extent the new responsibilities, which physicians gained in the 1760s, can be comparatively considered meaningful and useful.[24]

22 *Instruction För Kongl. Maj:ts Collegium Medicum ... 1763*, §§ 4–9.

23 On information gathering as a central cameralist practice, see Fors and Orrje, 'Describing the World,' 107–128.

24 Historian of science and medicine Gunnar Broberg tellingly sums up the contribution of what he calls 'Swedish Enlightenment medicine' as the creation of medical statistics, the building of hospitals, and the adoption of smallpox inoculation. Broberg, 'Liten svensk medicinhistoria,' 18.

Physicians inventing, advertising, and selling medicaments

The sale of medicaments was, like the practice of medicine, a highly contested area claimed by several groups of medical actors. Physicians and barber-surgeons were known to prepare medicines themselves, and to sell them directly to their patients. In places where there were no pharmacies nearby, town physicians or town barber-surgeons could take on the role of local apothecary as well. This was considered accepted practice. Furthermore, physicians serving the rural population often kept travel pharmacies, selling their contents directly to patients.[25] Indeed, a directive issued 12 April 1744, encouraged physicians' experimentation with medicaments, stating that, 'If [a] provincial doctor has knowledge of unknown medicaments [...] he shall let the apothecaries make them; but in such cases as he, with a clear conscience, can and wants to keep their manufacture a secret, he may prepare them himself, and give them to the apothecaries in his province to sell for a reasonable price. But he may not ply trade with them himself to the detriment of [the apothecaries].'[26] Selling medicaments was, unlike the medical practice of many a Swedish physician, a highly lucrative business. As remarked in the charming early eighteenth-century autobiography of the apothecary Johan Lambert,

> Our young Doctors on their journeys around the Academies in Europe want to learn to reason about everything, and to take degrees there cost the money of their parents, and then the heirs fight [to avoid paying] their student loans. [...] But would you not agree [...] is it not better at Pharmacies, less running about, and more gratitude, the patient comes to the counter by his own accord [...] and you bear no risk of contagion. [For this reason] we find that old, sly Doctors do not care to practice, but prefer to have, and to trade with, their own Chymical medicines, and arcana.[27]

One particularly sly doctor was Nils Rosén von Rosenstein (1706–1773). Although the son of a vicar, he would become well-connected in the highest echelons of society, gaining several prominent patients already as a young man in the 1730s. In 1734, he drew on contacts at the court to achieve election

25 Ahlberg, *Svenska farmaciens*, 80, 82.

26 *Kongl. Maj:ts Nådige Instruction ... 1744*, § 18. On the pan-European popularity of arcane medicines, see also Maehle, *Drugs on Trial*, 27.

27 Lambert attributes the words to one of his old masters. See Lambert, 'Johan Lamberts självbiografi,' 338–337.

to the Collegium Medicum and in 1735 he gained the title of physician to the king (Swe. *Kunglig Livläkare*).[28] Soon thereafter he became professor of medicine in Uppsala, but would resign from the chair some fifteen years later in order to move to Stockholm. A favourite of king Adolf Fredrik, Nils Rosén von Rosenstein was ennobled in 1762.[29]

Rosén's academic output was slight, but nevertheless he arguably established himself as eighteenth-century Sweden's most influential physician. Part of his fame rested on his publication of a great number of popular texts intended for a general audience. In particular, he published short medical essays in calendars (almanacs), beginning in 1737 and continuing until a few years before his death.[30] These calendars were undoubtedly Sweden's most important public venue for the dissemination of medical and scientific knowledge, especially after the Royal Swedish Academy of Science received the exclusive privilege to produce them. The year 1764 saw the publication of his most famous book, *Underrättelser om Barn-Sjukdomar*. An edited collection of essays previously published in calendars, it comprised an overview of, and suggested cures for, the most common maladies of children.[31]

Rosén's interest in pharmaceutical matters went back at least to 1735–36, when he lectured publicly in Uppsala on the *Pharmacopeja Holmiensis* and gave private instruction in *materia medica*. Later, he became well-known for his advocacy of chinchona bark as a cure for intermittent fevers, and created several pharmaceutical compositions, among them a widely known elixir, 'Roséns bröstdroppar.'[32] In 1765, he published his main pharmaceutical work, *Hus- och Reseapotek*. The booklet contained information about fifty-four medicaments deemed suitable for household use and for travelling purposes. Although the book states that the presented medicaments could be bought at pharmacies, the work was clearly also a companion volume to ready-made

28 For an overview of Rosén's early life and career, see Pehrsson. *Nils Rosén von Rosenstein*. Pehrsson covers Rosén's networks at 115–125, 146–149. Apparently, Rosén also had sex with one of his patients (see ibid.). It can also be mentioned that Abraham Bäck, the president of *Collegium Medicum* (1752–1795), belonged to the first generation of Rosén's students in Uppsala; see ibid., 129–131. See also Vahlquist and Wallgren, eds., *Nils Rosén von Rosenstein*. There exists a full-length biography of Rosén: see Sjögren, *Mannen*. It is however a hagiography of little discernible use for historians.

29 Lindroth, *Svensk Lärdomshistoria: Frihetstiden*, 476–478.

30 A bibliography of his works is found in Dintler 'Nils Rosén von Rosenstein. Bibliography,' 140–146.

31 Rosén von Rosenstein, *Underrättelser*. It would eventually be translated into several foreign languages and republished well into the nineteenth century. Vahlquist and Wallgren, eds., *Nils Rosén von Rosenstein*.

32 Nyström, *Nils Rosén von Rosenstein*.

pharmaceutical chests stocked with a set of the medicaments.[33] These chests were prepared by the apothecary Georgii of the Crown pharmacy (Swe. *Kronan*) in Stockholm. Testifying to their popularity, a great number of these chests still exist in Swedish collections.

Bottles and boxes in the Rosén–Georgii chests were labelled by numbers corresponding to the numbers given to the medicaments in Roséns book. Hence, it is clear that the chests and book were intended to be used together.[34] I have not yet ascertained whether Rosén was directly involved in the business of manufacturing the chest, or whether he perhaps received renumeration from the manufacturers. However, the medicine chests stocked by Georgii carried a printed label glued to the inside of the lid, which advertised the connection to Rosén.[35] Chests manufactured by the apothecary C. J. Sahlberg of the Moor pharmacy (Swe. *Morianen*, also in Stockholm) also appeared to have been stocked with the medicaments proposed by Rosén's book, and at least one remaining Sahlberg-manufactured chest, in a dedicated compartment, still contains an original copy of his booklet.[36]

The preparation of pharmaceutical chests for home and travel use was an established practice throughout Europe, and such chests were widely used by affluent travelers and housekeepers. Rosén's book was far from the first book on the subject to appear in the Swedish language. Hence, his book exploited an established market. But Rosén, the apothecaries who manufactured chests, and Collegium Medicum had additional audiences and other functions in mind. In the 1760s, Collegium Medicum tasked C. J. Sahlberg of the Moor pharmacy with creating compact models for portable home and travel pharmacies.[37] The initiative coincided with a reinstatement of the Collegium Medicum as the main agency of the state responsible for national public health issues. In 1766, when the Commission for Health was abolished, the responsibility of overseeing province physicians was handed over to the *Collegium*. In a revised directive for provincial doctors of the same year, it was specified that provincial doctors should be in possession

33 A pharmaceutical analysis of some of the compound medicaments in a historic Rosén medicine chest was made in 2019 by Hemström Trolin in *Cracking*.

34 I have inspected a number of medicine chests made from the seventeenth to the early nineteenth century at Nordiska Museet, which has about thirty, and Apotekarsocieteten, which possesses about fifteen.

35 *Hus- och rese- apoteque … tillagat på apotequet Kronan*. For an example of such a chest, see Gotlands Läns Museum, object id. GFDEP1453 http://samlingarna.gotlandsmuseum.se/index.php/Detail/objects/100717. Accessed 13 November 2021.

36 Axel-Nilsson, 'Ett hus- och rese-apoteque,' 144.

37 Lindeke 'Medicinkistor,' 10–11.

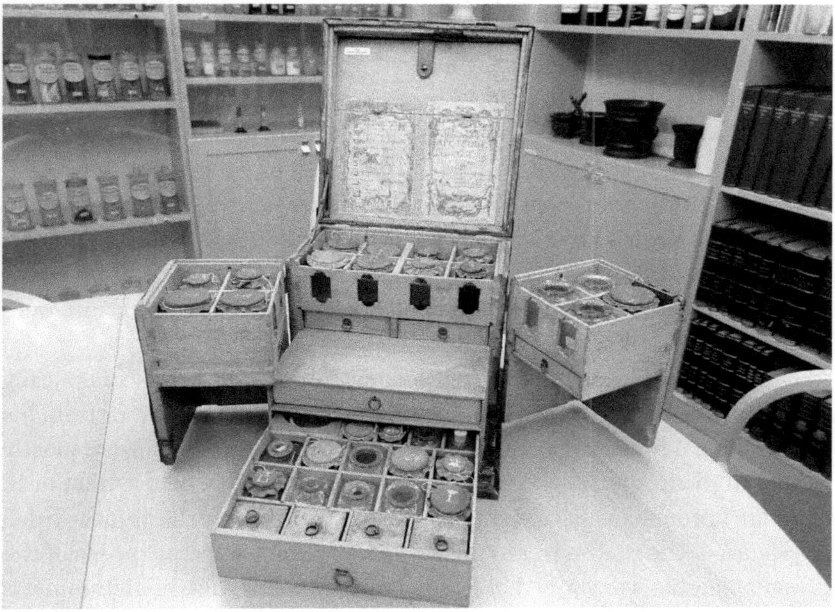

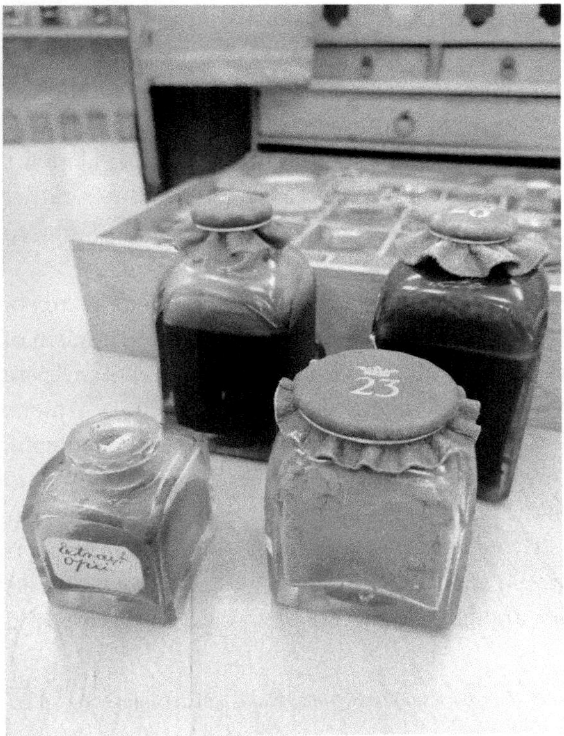

Figure 6.1 and 6.2. Figure 6.1 shows an opened Rosén–Georgii medicine chest with booklet, glued-in label, and original bottles and tins, many of which still contain the medicaments specified in the booklet. Figure 6.2 shows a selection of glass containers, three of which still have numeric label corresponding to entries in the booklet and serving also as the caps of the containers. From the collections of the Swedish Pharmaceutical Society (Swe. *Apotekarsocieteten*). The contents of some of the medicaments of this exceptionally well-preserved copy were analysed by Felix Hemström Trolin in 2019 as part of a master's thesis in pharmacognosy at Uppsala University. Photo: Felix Hemström Trolin.

of 'a suitable and well set-up pharmaceutical chest' (Swe: *tjenligt och wäl inrättadt Rese-Apotheque*). This directive was also renewed in 1774.[38]

The Rosén medicine chests thus had a ready market, which was furthermore well primed to receive them both through Rosén's published description of medicaments in the annual calendars, and through the efforts of the Collegium Medicum. It should, however, be noted that they faced stiff competition from other products of a similar nature. Such competitors included the home and travel pharmacies 'of Halle' (Swe. *Halliska hus- och reseapoteken*). Invented by the German physician C. F. Richter, from Halle, medicaments came with a book entitled *Erkentniss des Menschen*, and were sold both in pharmacies and in general stores.[39]

It remains to be ascertained to what extent Rosén benefitted economically from the production of the chests, from 'Roséns bröstdroppar' or from his other medical inventions. Be this as it may, perhaps benefits were mostly gained in the form of social capital, of which he already held a great deal. After all, Rosén managed to establish himself as probably the best-regarded physician of the realm. In any case, the key issue for the purposes of the present chapter is to show that Rosén's medicaments and medicine chests competed directly with the products of unlicensed practitioners, quacks, and mountebanks on the self-medication market. Many such products were secret and often exotically named remedies. The Rosén chests did not eschew marketing. It included elixirs with evocative names such as 'the Yellow Drops of the Prince,' Hoffman's White Drops' and 'Dr Durietz's Mother-Drops.' His descriptions of his medicines in the annual calendars perhaps should also be considered as advertisement for his products, rather than as an expression of disinterested and objective information, shared for the benefit of the public?

But before joining the chorus of eighteenth-century popular culture, in which a consistent theme was the ridicule, contempt, and skepticism of greedy physicians, we should recollect that self-interest and a genuine desire to improve society often went hand in hand for Enlightenment reformers. Being a physician to the king, a leading member of the Collegium Medicum, and a fellow of the Royal Swedish Academy of Sciences, Rosén seems not to have directly infringed on the privileges of apothecaries nor does he appear to have used his influence to directly seek to legally suppress his major competitors. Instead, it would appear that he used his extensive networks to cooperate with patrons and clients, medical and political actors, and

38 *Kongl. Maj:ts Nådiga Instruction … 1766*, § 12. *Kongl. Maj:ts Nådiga Instruction … 1774*, § 12.
39 Ahlberg, *Svenska farmaciens*, 96.

used the venues at his disposal to push for the medicaments and agendas he favored. The public good may indeed have been his main motivation.

In the discussion above, we have not touched upon the theoretical rationale behind eighteenth-century physicians proposed reforms of the pharmacopoeia. Rosén was active during a period of transition, which was characterised by a radical simplification of medicaments. This transition is highly visible in the sources. An illustration is provided by a comparison of the *Pharmacopoeia Svecica* of 1775, very much a product of Rosén's immediate circle of colleagues, with its predecessor the *Pharmacopoeja Holmiensis* (1686). The *Svecica* severely reduced both the number of listed compositions (recipes), and the number of ingredients used in compositions.[40] The work was part of a more general trend. The eighteenth century saw a gradual increase of use of medicaments that had specific physiological effects and targeted specific ailments. Chinchona-bark, which Rosén strongly advocated as a remedy for fevers, is one example. This rise in specificity was connected to the appearance and more widespread availability on Western markets of a varied set of exotic intoxicants – for example, coffee, tea, tobacco, cannabis, opium, and later heroin. Like alcohol, these drugs all had easily perceptible physiological effects. Moreover, the effect of one drug was comparably easy to distinguish from the effect of another, and individual drugs were often considered to have specific medicinal benefits. Many of these drugs were often used in elixirs, that is, they were dissolved in alcohol together with other ingredients. 'Roséns bröstdroppar' is as good an example as any of such an elixir. It consisted of opium, saffron, liquorice, and sugar dissolved in marsala wine. It was a simple and straightforward composition of up-to-date ingredients, all of which have perceptible physiological effects, depending on dosage.

The Rosén chests can clearly be described as part of an Enlightenment project that included an attempt by a physician to challenge quacks by enlisting the latest medical knowledge at his disposal. Indeed, the chests contained a standardised set of medicaments, manufactured to the highest standards, and validated by current medical theory and authorities. Importantly, the composition of the medicaments of the chests were public knowledge, and thus open to both scientific scrutiny and modification. Although such appreciative descriptions of eighteenth-century medicine have their merits, they are also woefully incomplete. Such positive appraisals ignore complexity by focusing on physicians' medical practices that appear to be forward-looking while ignoring practices that seem to be old-fashioned or

40 For an overview of this transition, see Ahlberg, *Svenska farmaciens*, 354–355.

strange. They also drive a wedge between physicians and other practitioners, thus ignoring the methodological symmetry criteria (see the introduction to this chapter), which provides a more complex critical assessment.

Sofia Ling, in a study of the relationship between licensed and unlicensed medical practitioners in Sweden between 1770 and 1870, points out that although the term *quack* is now very negatively laden, it need not necessarily to have been so historically.[41] Quacks, furthermore, could be difficult to distinguish from householders, married women, and others who cared for sick relatives, friends, and neighbours, often composing and administering their self-prepared remedies and cures. There was an enormous wealth of such cures and medicaments that were shared, sold, and exchanged by people at all levels of society: from queens and counts, to farmers and poor cottage dwellers. Rosén was not the only influential physician who collected and made compendia of useful house remedies. Indications are that many physicians were curious and respectful to the knowledge, cures, and medicines of other medical actors. A foreign surgeon, a poor old lady in a cottage, or a travelling mountebank could, potentially, have access to and administer excellent cures or medicines.[42]

Physicians were never regarded as the sole source of the best medical care. Throughout the eighteenth century, patients regarded experience and a good track record as superior indicators of an effective healer. Formal exams and titles were of less importance. There are indications in the source material that many physicians shared this view. The sharp distinction between licensed and unlicensed practitioners, which is visible in legal documents such as charters, did not always correspond to everyday reality. As we have seen, the legal measures available to physicians were few, and patients could always go elsewhere. It should also be noted that the Swedish rural population was literate to a rather high degree. Hence they, too, could access recent medical literature. When in 1775, the rural healer Lars Larsson was called upon by his local church council of Ljusnarberg to explain his alleged superstitious practices, he responded by producing three published works on medicine. A Swedish translation of Elias Beynon the younger's *The Good Samarian* (first published in German in 1663), a copy of Frantz Michael von Aken's *House and Travel Pharmacy* (1746) and Johan Anders af Darelli's *Parish Pharmacy and House Remedies* (1760 or 1771). He also

41 On average the *Collegium* examined two to three cases per year, or 282 cases for the whole of the period studied (1770–1889). Ling, *Kärringmedicin*, 12, 16, 23–24, 69, 77.

42 Ling, *Kärringmedicin*, 141–145; Tillhagen, *Folklig läkekonst*, 1–2, 54–55; Lindroth, *Svensk Lärdomshistoria: Frihetstiden*, 418.

explained that he had access to two more medical books at home, and that he bought his medical supplies in licensed pharmacies. His performance was apparently so impressive that several members of the church council were prepared to vouch that Lars Larsson was an honest and sensible man (Swe. *beskedlig man*).[43]

The healer Lars Larsson thus held an excellent performance in demonstrating his medical credibility. But just as Larsson knew how to present his knowledge in the correct framework of (roughly) contemporary medical knowledge, elite practitioners could adopt the language of quackery and promote the high hopes of miracle cures that came with it. Secret remedies of various types were often highly regarded both by the general population and influential physicians. Rosén, when he stepped down from the presidency of the Royal Swedish Academy of Sciences in 1746, lamented the many effective medical treatments that had been kept secret and consequently had been lost with the death of their inventors.[44] These were not empty words. In their role as knowledge-holders in the field of medicine, physicians could be used by the state to give advice. To further blur the line between unlicensed and licensed practitioners, let me conclude this essay with a short narrative of Rosén's involvement in vouching for and procuring an English secret remedy for the benefit of the Swedish state.

The following anecdote is an informative example of the procurement of a mysterious medication, allegedly a successful remedy for cancer. Such a medicament was bought by the Swedish state from London surgeon Richard Guy.[45] The remedy became known to the Swedish travelling medical student Pehr Bjerchén during his stay in England in 1758. Bjerchén promptly promoted it in letters to at least two of the most influential Swedish physicians of the day, Rosén and Abraham Bäck. The former was quickly convinced of its efficacy. It should be bought by the Swedish state and used for the benefit of its citizens. Rosén contacted a patron in the government, the Chancellor of the Realm Carl Fredrik Scheffer. Scheffer acted promptly to secure the remedy. It turned out that the secret recipe itself was not for sale, but after some negotiations, it was agreed in 1759 that the Commission for Health would be permitted to buy the knowledge of how to use it, and receive a supply whenever it was needed for a period of twenty-five years.

43 Tillhagen, *Folklig läkekonst*, 55. The editions given below and in the bibliography are the latest Swedish editions available at the time. But Larsson may well have owned earlier editions than these: von Aken, *Hus- och rese-apotheque*; Beynon, Gufer, and Coler, *Then barmhertige samariten*; Darelli, *Socken apothek och några hus-curer.*

44 Rosén, *Tal om en opartisk*, 41–42.

45 There are six further examples in Ahlberg, *Den Svenska farmaciens*, 97–101.

The keeper of the secret knowledge of how to use it properly would be Pehr Bjerchén, the intermediary who negotiated the purchase. The purchase price was the exceptional sum of 3,000 pounds sterling! What prompted this swift action? Historian of medicine Otto Hjelt suggests that Rosén acted to secure the remedy together with the Councillor of the Realm Karl Gustaf Löwenhielm, who was another of his patrons, for whom Rosén acted as a family doctor. The remedy was probably procured as a final desperate attempt to save Löwenhjelm's dying wife, Juliana Constantia. The cure, however, arrived too late. Madame Löwenhielm died just a few days after Bjerchén's return with the medicament from England. The death of Madame Löwenhielm was, however, not blamed on Bjerchén, nor was the remedy's efficacy discredited. Bjerchén would continue to use it with much success in his medical practice until his death in 1774. Thus, Bjerchén's dealing in arcane medicaments were highly beneficial for his career, and it can be noted that he both became a member of the Collegium Medicum and eventually was ennobled af Bjerkén, in 1773.[46] The Bjerchén example demonstrates how Sweden's most prominent physicians were more than ready to trust, and place all their professional influence behind a secret remedy, invented by a foreigner and non-physician. If Hjelt's interpretation is correct, this example also reveals how officials in different parts of the state apparatus called in favors and drew on personal networks to divert state resources for private purposes.[47] Thus the story well illustrates my theses that physicians were not as aloof from other medical practitioners as the often have been portrayed, and that they permitted loyalty to patrons and patients to trump their construction of professional identity.

Conclusions

The aim of this chapter has been to revise inherited notions and traditional historiography with regards to the role of physicians in eighteenth-century Swedish society. I have argued that we should leave aside the notion of the comparably high status of physicians, and instead consider them as one group of actors among many on a medical market. Physicians had to relate

46 Hjelt, *Svenska statens*, 1–28.

47 Such schemes were not uncommon during the eighteenth century. Although clearly corrupt by today's standards, this was not as clear-cut during the eighteenth century. Early modern rulers and politicians were often expected to redistribute state resources to clients to keep them loyal.

and negotiate their positions and activities with other medical actors who occupied partly different and partly overlapping market niches. Actual medical, social, and economic practice should be distinguished from the cameralist and Enlightenment rhetoric which physicians used to ingratiate themselves with elites as well as to strengthen their hand against competing groups who provided medical care. Thus, it is quite possible to account for the enlightening and improvement-oriented activities of eighteenth-century Swedish physicians as examples of profit-seeking and networking within the framework of a patriotic, improvement-oriented discourse, which was a mainstay during the Swedish Age of Liberty.[48] That physicians adopted such language and practices is therefore to be expected. That they did so successfully should also not come as a surprise. They were, to a certain extent, courtiers providing advice on personal health. Similarly, that their advice on other issues would be heeded should also come as no surprise. But historians should not take such persuasive rhetoric at face value. Other factors ought to be acknowledged. Influential and famous physicians, such as Abraham Bäck, Nils Rosén von Rosenstein, and Carl Linnaeus, established themselves as clients of leading politicians in the highest echelons of power. They also connected vertically with actors in other corporations and organisations.

However, the existence of such activities and affiliations does not imply that physicians, or their organisations, had important functions in the state, or that they directed public health policies in any meaningful way. Instead, we must acknowledge that physicians were active in several arenas, and in many contexts, but that they acted mostly as patrons and clients, rather than as representatives of a collective, or corporation of physicians. We should not focus only on formal, corporative organisations such as the Collegium Medicum, but perhaps instead look with greater peripheral vision at how individual physicians acted in other arenas – for example, the politically appointed commissions, and the Diet, which when assembled, became an important arena for building the informal networks that lay beneath and supported institutionalisation. Another important arena was the Royal Swedish Academy of Sciences, where society's elite met and mingled with knowledge-holders placed at various locations, and in various organisations that were connected to the state to a stronger or weaker degree.

Furthermore, I have argued that physicians' connection to the state remained tenuous throughout the eighteenth century. The connections that did exist depended more on personal networks of individual physicians than on formal organisations such as the *Collegium Medicum*. Indeed, it

48 See n. 5.

seems that from the point of view of public health, the services that physicians could provide were rather unimportant throughout the eighteenth century. Thus, physicians, as a group, should not be considered essentially different from other groups of health providers on the medical market, such as travelling quacks, countryside healers, midwives, barber-surgeons, dentists, apothecaries, and bathers.

This said, the authority of physicians, and the Collegium Medicum, gradually increased over the century. However, unlike other state officials bearing the title of *assessors*, physicians mostly managed their own professional interests. In this respect, their corporation bears a greater resemblance to a guild (e.g., the guild of hatters) than to the other state bureaus of the Swedish civil service. It can be noted that when the Collegium finally was assigned a few, new formal duties in the mid-1760s, it began proposing programs of reform of a type which had been in action in the official branches of the Swedish state for at least sixty years. It is also unclear what legacy can be attributed to the reforms and activities of the Collegium Medicum. The legal framework for Collegium Medicum's policing of the health of the realm would survive the Age of Liberty. The 1763 directives were reissued once more in 1774, which in very similar formulations mirrored the previous one.[49] Although programmes were not abandoned outright, medical reforming zeal nevertheless waned quickly in the following decades. Foreign interest in the Swedish example, which had been a feature of the Age of Liberty, was also waning. Towards the final decades of the century, many ideas about public health reform were summarised and expounded by a German, Johann Peter Frank (1745–1821). He coined the phrase 'medical policing' (Ger. *medicinischen Polizey*) and his work became an inspiration for later state-directed regulatory efforts regarding social medicine and hygiene.[50] Simultaneously, there is no denying that the partially successful attempt of the Collegium to transform physicians into officials, responsible for enforcing rules and regulations, should be seen as a cameralist, or perhaps Enlightenment project. It also gave physicians a measure of formal influence and official status. But this chapter points to the patchy and partial nature of narratives that depict eighteenth-century institutionalisation and reform

49 *Kongl. Maj:ts Nådiga instruction ... 1774*. The King's interest in further medical reforms would, however, prove to be small. Sandblad, *Världens nordligaste*, 16.

50 Qvarsell, *Vårdens idéhistoria*, 36–37. An overview of the state of Swedish public health towards the end of the eighteenth century is given in Schultz von Schultzenheim, *Tal om den offentliga vården, ... 1799*, 83–103, 113–211.

within the Swedish medical market. They rarely reflect the realities of practice and are, to a certain extent, artefacts of an over-reliance on institutional archives, as well as projections of later developments onto earlier historical events.

Bibliography

Printed works

Beynon, Elias, Johann Gufer, and Johann Coler. *Then barmhertige samariten, thet är: Wälment råd och vnderrättelse, huruledes man allahanda menniskians in- och vtwärtes siukdomar och bräckligheter med ringa, oansenliga, doch godfundna läkedomar hielpa kan, them fattigom, och särdeles på landet boendom, til nytto och gagn beskrifwit af Elias Beynon then yngre ; samt ett kort vttog af Johan Guffers lilla Hus-apothek af samma innehåll ; sidst en liten husläkedom af tobak ; item, Coleri vnderwisning om hälsones förwahring i hwar månad om åhret; ther jemte ett nödigt register.* Stockholm: Horrn, 1727.

Darelli, Johan Anders af. *Socken apothek och några hus-curer, utgifne under kongl: collegii medici öfwerseende och besörjande. Andra uplagan något förbättrad.* Stockholm: Stolpe, 1771.

Hus- och rese- apoteque på hennes Kongl. Majts, nådigste befallning inrättat af wälborne herr archiatern och riddaren, Rosén von Rosenstein, tillagat på apotequet Kronan af Georgii. Printed label on pharmaceutical travelling chest in the collections of Apotekarsocieteten, Stockholm.

Instruction För Kongl. Maj:ts Collegium Medicum, såsom nödig tilläggning uti 1688 års Medicinal-Ordning, i anledning af the sidstledne Riksdag hos Kongl. Maj:t gjorde underdåniga erhindringar til Medicinal-Wärkets uphielpande i Riket. Skrifwen Stockholm i Råd-Cammaren then 22 Junii 1763. Stockholm: Kongl. Tryckeriet, 1763.

Kongl. Maj:ts Nådiga Instruction för Provincial-Medici, Gifwen Ekolsund then 29 Julii 1774. 1774.

Kongl. Maj:ts Nådiga Instruction, Hwarefter the Provincial Doctorer, som af Kronan eller någon Publique Fond njuta någon wiss och ständig lön, hafwa sig at rätta. Skrifwen Stockholm i Råd-Cammaren then 18 November 1766. Stockholm: Kongl. Tryckeriet, 1766.

Kongl. Maj:ts Nådige Instruction Hwarefter The Provincial Doctorer, som af Cronan eller på Städernes Stater niuta någon wiss och ständig Lön, hafwa sig at rätta. Skrifwen Stockholm i Råd-Cammaren then 12. April 1744. Stockholm: Kongl. Tryckeriet, 1744.

Rosén von Rosenstein, Nils. *Tal om en opartisk och förnuftig medici förnämsta göromål, hållit för Kongl. Svenska Vetenskapskaademien af… Nils Rosén då han afträdde sit praesidium d. 12 april 1746.* Stockholm: Lars Salvius, 1746.

Rosén von Rosenstein, Nils. *Underrättelser om Barn-Sjukdomar och deras Bote-Medel: tillförene styckewis utgifne uti de små Almanachorna, nu samlade, tilökte och förbättrade.* Stockholm: Lars Salvius, 1764.

Schultz von Schultzenheim, David. *Tal om den offentliga vården, i hänseende till folkets seder och helsa, samt de fattigas lifbergning, hållet för K:gl Svenska Vetenskaps-Academien … den 30 januarii, år 1799.* Stockholm: Joh. P. Lindh, 1801.

von Aken, Frantz Michaël. *Hus- och rese-apotheque, huru man sin hälsa rätt skjöta, och the rätta approberade medel, vti ett hushåll, bruka skal, vti möjeligaste kortthet sammandragit.* Skara: Herm. Arnold Moeller, 1746.

Literature

Ahlberg, Karl. *Den Svenska farmaciens historia.* Stockholm: Billes, 1908.

Axel-Nilsson, Christian. 'Ett hus- och rese-apoteque.' In *Fataburen: Nordiska museet och Skansens årsbok*, 142–144. Stockholm: Nordiska Museet, 1962.

Bloor, David. *Knowledge and Social Imagery.* 2nd ed. Chicago: University of Chicago Press, 1991.

Broberg, Gunnar. 'Liten svensk medicinhistoria.' In *Til at stwdera läkedom: Tio studier I svensk medicinhistoria*, edited by G. Broberg, 9–50. Lund: Sekel, 2008.

Cavallin, Maria. *I kungens och folkets tjänst: Synen på den svenske ämbetsmannen 1750–1780.* Gothenburg: Göteborgs universitet, 2003.

Dintler, Åke. 'Nils Rosén von Rosenstein. Bibliography.' In *Nils Rosén von Rosenstein and his Textbook on Paediatrics*, edited by Bo Vahlquist and Arvid Wallgren, 140–146. Uppsala: Almqvist & Wiksell, 1964.

Fors, Hjalmar. '"Away! Away to Falun!": J. G. Gahn and the Application of Enlightenment Chemistry to Smelting.' *Technology and Culture* 50, no. 3 (2009): 549–568.

Fors, Hjalmar. *The Limits of Matter: Chemistry, Mining and Enlightenment.* Chicago: University of Chicago Press, 2015.

Fors, Hjalmar. 'Matematiker mot linneaner: Konkurrerande vetenskapliga nätverk kring Torbern Bergman.' In *Vetenskapens sociala strukturer: Sju historiska fallstudier om konflikt, samverkan och makt*, edited by S. Widmalm, 25–53. Lund: Nordic Academic Press, 2008.

Fors, Hjalmar. 'Medicine and the Making of a City: Spaces of Pharmacy and Scholarly Medicine in Seventeenth-Century Stockholm.' *Isis* 107, no. 3 (2016): 473–494.

Fors, Hjalmar, and Jacob Orrje. 'Describing the World and Shaping the Self: Knowledge-Gathering, Mobility and Spatial Control at the Swedish Bureau of Mines.' In *Transnational Culture of Expertise: Circulating State Related Knowledge in the 18th and 19th Centuries*, edited by J. Vogel and L. Schilling, 107–128. Berlin: De Gruyter Oldenbourg, 2019.

Fritz, Martin. 'Göteborg under det sena 1700-talet – avkrok eller inkörsport?' In *Ljus över landet?: Upplysningen som drivkraft i 1700-talets svenska vetenskap och vitterhet*, edited by P. Hallberg. Gothenburg: Kungl. Vetenskaps- och Vitterhetssamhället i Göteborg, 2005.

Gustafsson, Tony. *Läkaren, döden och brottet: Studier i den svenska rättsmedicinens etablering*. Uppsala: Uppsala universitet, 2007.

Hemström Trolin, Felix. *Cracking Hundreds of Years Old Pharmaceutical Trade Secrets; A Study of the 18th Century Medicinal Chest of Physician Nils Rosén von Rosenstein*. Research Project in Pharmacognosy, 30 hp. Supervisor: Nils-Otto Ahnfelt. Fall semester, 2019.

Hjelt, Otto E. A. *Svenska och finska medicinalverkets historia 1663–1812*. 3 vols. Helsinki: Helsingfors Centraltryckeri, 1891–1893.

Hjelt, Otto E. A. *Svenska statens inköp af hemliga läkemedel, och särskildt kirurgen Guy's medel mot kräfta*. Helsinki: Finska Litteratursällskapets tryckeri, 1888.

Hodacs, Hanna, and Kenneth Nyberg. *Naturalhistoria på resande fot: om att forska, undervisa och göra karriär i 1700-talets Sverige*. Lund: Nordic Academic Press, 2007.

Kock, Wolfram, ed. *Medicinalväsendet I Sverige 1813–1962: Utgiven med anledning av Kungl. Medicinalstyrelsens 300-årsjubileum*. Stockholm: Nordiska Bokhandeln, 1963.

Lambert, Johan. 'Johan Lamberts självbiografi.' In *Sveriges Apotekarhistoria: Från konung Gustaf I:s till närvarande tid*, vol. 1., edited by A. Levertin, C. F. V. Schimmelpfennig & K. A. Ahlberg, 324–54. Stockholm: Ernst Westerberg, 1910–1918.

Lindeke, Björn. 'Medicinkistor, hus-, rese- och sockenapotek.' *Unicornis* 1 (2013): 10–11.

Lindroth, Sten. *Svensk Lärdomshistoria: Frihetstiden*. Södertälje: Norstedts, 1989.

Ling, Sofia. *Kärringmedicin och vetenskap: Läkare och kvacksalverianklagade i Sverige omkring 1770–1870*. Uppsala: Uppsala universitet, 2004.

Maehle, Andreas Holger. *Drugs on Trial: Experimental Pharmacology and Therapeutic Innovation in the Eighteenth Century*. Amsterdam: Rodopi, 1999.

Nyström, Eva. 'Nils Rosén von Rosenstein.' *Svenskt biografiskt lexikon*, urn:sbl:6892. https://sok.riksarkivet.se/sbl/artikel/6892. Accessed 11 October 2021.

Orrje, Jacob. *Mechanicus: Performing an Early Modern Persona*. Uppsala: Uppsala universitet, 2015.

Paulsson Holmberg, Tove. *Onaturlig födelse: Johan von Hoorn och det obstetriska dilemma 1680–1730*. Lund: Lunds universitet, 2017.

Pehrsson, Anna-Lena. *Nils Rosén von Rosenstein en medicinhistorisk biografi över åren 1706–1740*. Uppsala: Uppsala universitet, 2006.

Qvarsell, Roger. *Vårdens idéhistoria*. Stockholm: Carlssons, 1991.

Sandblad, Henrik. *Världens nordligaste läkare: Medicinalväsendets första insteg i Nordskandinavien 1750–1810*. Stockholm: Almqvist & Wiksell, 1979.

Sjögren, Iréne. *Mannen som förlängde livet: Nils Rosén von Rosenstein*. Stockholm: Carlssons, 2006.

Tillhagen, Carl-Herman. *Folklig läkekonst*. Stockholm: LTs Förlag, 1962.

Vahlquist, Bo, and Arvid Wallgren, eds. *Nils Rosén von Rosenstein and his Textbook on Paediatrics*. Uppsala: Almqvist & Wiksell, 1964.

Vainio-Korhonen, Kirsi. *De frimodiga: Barnmorskor, födande och kroppslighet på 1700-talet*. Translated by Camilla Frostell. Helsinki: Svenska litteratursällskapet i Finland, 2016.

Widenberg, Johanna. *Den stora kreatursdöden: Kampen mot boskapspest och mjältbrand I 1700-talets svenska rike*. Stockholm: Carlssons, 2017.

Windahl Pontén, Annika. *Kiär hustru, wackra barn, bodde I ett palais: Identitet och materialitet i hushållet Linné*. Uppsala: Uppsala universitet, 2020.

About the Author

Hjalmar Fors is a historian of the history of science and ideas. He is Head of Unit at the Hagströmer Medico-Historical Library, Karolinska Institutet. His primary research interests include the history of early modern empirical sciences, in particular the history of chemistry, alchemy, pharmacy, medicine and natural history.

8. Gender, Health, and Hair in Sweden, 1740–1840

Hedvig Widmalm

Abstract
This chapter examines changing views on haircare, health, and gender in Sweden from 1740 to 1840. By investigating haircare in recipes, journals, and advertising, the chapter outlines the connections drawn between outer appearances and inner wellness in the early modern period. It also shows how these connections were gendered. In the eighteenth century, hair was commercialised through the use of wigs and a growing market for haircare recipes. These recipes were a mixture of health cures and cosmetic concoctions. By the early nineteenth century, haircare manuals were becoming more gendered than before. Books about haircare for men were focused on hair as a signifier of health, while haircare and advertising for women was concerned with hair as a signifier of beauty.

Keywords: health, beauty, haircare, medicine, gender, bodies

Introduction

This chapter examines the connections between haircare, medicine, gender, and health in Sweden between the years 1740 and 1840. The periodisation covers a drastic change in hair fashions, particularly for elite men who went from wearing powdered hairstyles and wigs in the eighteenth century to more moderate styles in the early nineteenth century. It also covers the growth of a type of literature about haircare and cosmetics, a genre that was separate from but which still drew on household recipes and medical texts. Advice literature, newspapers, and journals of this period created a discursive framework in which beauty tips were combined with popular conceptions of medical science. In these diverse texts, hair was a part of the

Eyice, M. and C. Forss (eds.), *Health and Society in Early Modern Sweden.*
Taylor & Francis Group 2024
DOI 10.5117/9789463724296_CH08

body and thus a signifier of a body's health, vitality, and morality. At the same time, hair was something separate, easy to alter, remove, and transform into a commodity. Moreover, it was paradoxically both gendered and not gendered. By comparing different genres of writing, this chapter shows that there was a tension between the various ways hair was conceptualised during this period. One continuous strand in the discussions of hair and haircare throughout the period is the connection drawn between healthy hair and health of the body.

The chapter includes an overview of the way haircare appeared in economic texts, medical writing, popular journals, and haircare manuals. The study additionally examines the growth of a new genre of advice literature in Sweden, and how it carried with it traditions from older genres. The purpose of this critical inquiry is to answer the questions: How was hair related to health in different kinds of texts between 1740 and 1840? How and when was haircare medicalised, and for whom? And finally, what does this say about the relations between gender, health, and hair throughout this period?

A history of hair in Europe, from the mid-seventeenth to the early nineteenth century

In the early modern period, hair was both an intrinsic part of the body and something separate from it. This was an example of how physicians and scientists understood the physical nature of humans according to competing and concurrent theories of how the human body worked. At this time, the European scientific community was exploring a way to understand the human body as a machine. In 1703, the Dutch physician Herman Boerhaave gave lectures in medicine in which he described the sick body as similar to a clock with defective parts that only a skilled clockmaker, a physician, could repair.[1] In 1747, the French physician Julien Offray de La Mettrie published the groundbreaking work *L'homme machine*, partly influenced by seventeenth-century debates about whether animals had souls or if they were like machines.[2] However, despite these new works, the Roman philosopher Galen's (c. 129–c. 216 CE) ancient theory of humours was still accepted within the medical field and would remain so well into the nineteenth century. According to this theory, the body consisted of a balance

1 Wright, 'Metaphysics and Physiology,' 256.

2 Thomson, 'Animals, Humans, Machines,' 4, 36–37. See also La Mettrie and Thomson, *Machine Man and Other Writings*.

of four humours: yellow bile, blood, phlegm, and black bile. These humours were connected to the qualities of hot, cold, wet, and dry. In antiquity, the theory of humours was used mainly to understand the physical makeup of bodies, but in the Middle Ages, humours became connected to different forms of temperament: choleric, sanguine, phlegmatic, and melancholic.[3] Different bodies were assumed to possess different balances of humours. For example, female bodies were considered colder and wetter, while male bodies were hotter and drier. Galen's theory also explained the way human hair grew, what colour it was, and whether it was strong or weak. Hair was understood to absorb moisture from the body as it grew, and the nature of this moisture determined its colour, shape, and strength. The colour showed the temperament of the human. If that temperament was hot, it scorched the hair black, while yellow or white hair, associated with young children and the elderly, was the sign of phlegmatic weakness. The heat and dryness of male bodies was also seen as the reason why men were more prone to lose their scalp hair than women.[4] This did not explain why men had an abundance of facial hair and body hair compared to women. Still, despite its inconsistencies, Galen's theory of humours was the physiological theory most cited in writings about hair in the early modern period.

Despite the fact that humoral theories espoused the close and innate connection between hair and the character of the bodies they came from, hair became a commodity. Hair was used in the creation of elaborate so-called *allonge*-wigs, an aristocratic fashion that began in France at the court of Louis XIII (1601–1643).[5] Though wigs began as a fashion for the elite, by the mid-eighteenth century, the wig had ceased to be an exclusive marker of the nobility and different wigs instead became associated with different professions.[6] Consequently wigmaker guilds gradually became numerous in France. This commodification of hair coincided with an expansion of medical science, which meant that the human body was examined and charted in ways that had previously not been possible. The scientific revolution permitted people to study hair closely, to determine whether and how the body it came from affected the hair's quality. The scientist Anthony Van Leeuwenboek put a strand of hair under the microscope in 1678 and concluded that it was hollow in shape. This meant that it could be presumed

3 Grant 'Steiner and the Humours,' 57–58, 60; Singer, *Galen,* x–xi. On humoral theories in a Swedish context, see the chapters by Gabriela Bjarne Larsson, Charlotta Forss, Andreas Hellerstedt, and Anton Runesson in this volume.

4 Snook, 'Beautiful Hair, Health, and Privilege,' 26–28, 31.

5 Powell, 'Class and Social Status,' 159.

6 Kwass, 'Big Hair,' 634–639, 657.

to absorb nutrients and change depending on environmental conditions. This discovery went against the understanding that hair was exclusively affected by the body's balance of humours.[7] It also had commercial implications for a burgeoning market. If hairs were hollow, they could be receptive to hair treatments. If they were not intimately connected to the bodies they came from, they could be bought and sold, and made into wigs. However, as mentioned, different scientific theories on the body coexisted throughout the eighteenth century, and manuals on hairdressing continued to use humoral theories to define hair and prescribe treatments.[8] Problems that plagued hair were also discussed in the scientific community, not least, whether these problems were caused by scurvy, venereal disease, and/or head lice.[9]

The fashion for wigs spread from France to other nations. In Sweden, a guild for wigmakers was formed in 1664. As wigs became more widely adopted in the 1730s, the crown issued several tracts regulating the buying and selling of hair in its attempt to curb the import of hair from abroad as part of the protectionist trade policies of this period.[10] One commercial reason why the wig fashion continued into the eighteenth century was that the wigmakers' guilds were invested in promoting the practice.[11]

It should be noted that in Sweden, where more than 90 per cent of the population belonged to the farming sector, French fashions were still associated with members of the elite. Especially when it came to women, elaborate hairstyles were the privilege of the aristocracy and a small group of urban burghers. Most farmers' wives and widows covered their hair with close-fitting caps or shawls. Sumptuary laws give an indication of who pursued new French trends by showing which groups could be penalised. These regulations were not directed at the farming population until the very end of the eighteenth century, meaning that their consumption of new fashions only became noteworthy in this period.[12]

Though England and France were leaders in European fashions during the eighteenth century, this does not mean their fashions were adopted

7 Markiewicz, 'Hair, Wigs and Wig-Wearing,' 49; Corson, *Fashions in Hair*, 272; Rowland (translated by Fågelberg), *Filosofisk och praktisk afhandling*, 6, 13.

8 Markiewicz, 'Hair, Wigs and Wig-Wearing,' 52–53; Rosenthal, 'Raising Hair,' 1.

9 Powell and Roach, 'Health and Hygiene,' 92, 97.

10 See the pamphlets 'Publication Angående Bönhaseri'; 'Ytterligare Kungörelse Och Förbud'; Kungörelse, at ej någon må med Hårs friserande.'

11 Corson, *Fashions in Hair*, 265, 269.

12 Runefelt, *Att Hasta mot undergången*, 239; Rahikainen and Vainio-Korhonen, in Nyberg and Wachenfeldt, eds., 'Manlig och kvinnlig lyx,' 28–36.

wholesale in other countries. Aside from the economic and morally tinged criticisms against them as a wasteful foreign influence, there was some public criticism in Sweden about the way French hair fashions impacted public health. Critics in the journal *Stockholms-Posten* noted the fact that French fashions were not adapted to the cold Nordic climate and thus posed a health hazard.[13] Medical science of that time stressed the importance of keeping the body at a stable temperature.[14] As this chapter will show, wigs, powders, and pomades were also subject to criticism for the effects they were presumed to have on the heads of their wearers.

Beyond these above-mentioned concerns, there were other reasons why wig fashions fell out of favour. Wigs became less popular in all of Europe after the French revolution, which was part of a general rejection of fashions connected to the *ancien régime*.[15] With the imposition of new taxes on hair powder, the wig was also phased out for economic reasons.[16] The wig fashion's disappearance did not mean that haircare stopped being a matter of public concern however. In Sweden, a new genre of literature exclusively about haircare emerged in the nineteenth century. Most of these works were in fact not new, but they were translated to Swedish for the first time. Many of them also drew connections between health and haircare. However, though the genre was new, the connections between haircare and medicine were not. They were apparent in other, older forms of literature and laid the groundwork for this genre.

Hair and household: moral, economic and scientific justifications for haircare in the eighteenth century

An early Swedish instruction book *Kårt och redig Underwisning om Färge-Konsten* (Short and orderly instruction on the art of dyeing), included a longer section about cosmetic haircare. Published in 1747, it contained recipes for dyeing cloths, and for dyeing hair. As with many books of similar genres from this period, it claimed to be a translation and the original author was not listed. However, the short introduction had a clear ideological theme,

13 *Stockholms-posten*, 25 April 1788, 1.

14 Markiewicz, 'Hair, Wigs and Wig-Wearing,' 61. For a parallel discussion of this, see Charlotta Forss's chapter in this volume.

15 Laver, *Costume and Fashion*, 153; Oldstone-Moore, *Of Beards and Men*, 149; Kwass, 'Big Hair,' 647, 652, 659; Festa, 'Personal Effects,' 74–75.

16 Festa, 'Personal Effects,' 81–82; Kwass, 'Big Hair,' 659; Corson, *Fashions in Hair*, 276.

namely that these arts had been studied by learned men of science, and that they would be useful to 'fäderneslandet,' the fatherland.[17]

A religious and patriotic ideology was predominant in the Swedish kingdom at this time. It drew a connection between the kingdom, *fäderneslandet*, and the notion of the ideal household. This is a concept necessary to explore, even in relation to something as seemingly frivolous as haircare, as it was closely connected to scientific developments in the eighteenth century. It shows how cosmetic remedies for hair could be legitimised as something both scientific and economically sound to pursue.

During this period, the subject of economics was called either 'oeconomie' or 'hushållning,' housekeeping. Households were not private homes, but workplaces where people collaborated and constantly moved in and out.[18] The subject of 'housekeeping' was therefore wider in scope than the modern field of economics because it was embedded in culture, and because it had moral and religious connotations. *Hushållning* was an way of understanding a diverse set of housekeeping practices, influenced by the notion of divine hierarchical order of the household described in Martin Luther's catechism as well as the Aristotelian notion of the ideal *oikos*.[19] In the eighteenth century, scientists, economists, physicians, and housekeepers published practical advice through manuals, medicine books, and cookbooks, ostensibly to help common Swedish and Finnish farmers manage their households in accordance with this doctrine. From the points of view of contemporary scientists, housekeeping was the discovery and utilising of the gifts of nature that God provided to their fullest potential. The botanist Carl Linneaus's acolyte Elias Aspelin expressed this idea in the foreword to his book *Flora Oeconomica, Eller Hushålls-Nyttan af de I Swerige Wildt wäxande Örter* (Flora Oeconomica, or the Household's uses of Sweden's wild-growing herbs):

> To rightly understand and utilise something, is a science, that is as useful as it is indispensable, for which reason man, in whose service all of nature exists, is obliged to carefully get to know the nature and quality of created things, utilise them to their full utility, and to finally sensibly therefore praise the Originator on his own and all of Nature's behalf.[20]

17 Anonymous author, *Kårt och redig Underwisning*, i–ii.

18 Ågren, 'Introduction: Making a Living,' 7–8; Lindström et al., 'Working Together,' 61.

19 Frängsmyr, 'Den gudomliga ekonomin,' 218; Runefelt, *Hushållningens dygder*, 25, 92–93, 100–101; Lindström and Hassan Jansson, 'Pigan i fadersväldet,' 372; Harvey, *The Little Republic*, ch. 1; Lindberg, *Praemia et poenae*, 222.

20 Aspelin, *Flora Oeconomica*, Introduction.

The foreword emphasised the usefulness of each plant described, and that making use of them was a way to praise the Originator, God. In this book, 'Pinguicula' or 'Tätört' is described as a plant that could be used as a pomade and hair lightening treatment.[21] Today, an old name for this plant is 'hair-yellow' (Swe. *hårgula*), indicating that it was once used for the purpose Aspelin described.[22] The book contained advice on how to use flowers and herbs for various medical treatments and fly-poison, as well as for decoration and makeup. So there was room in this book for practical, decorative, and cosmetic uses of plants. The unifying theme was 'Oeconomia,' the economy of the household. Plants were useful for the individual household and moreover, all the book's named plants could be found within the borders of the Swedish realm, which was considered the nation's household.

Aspelin's book was based heavily on Carl Linneaus's own research. As Annika Windahl Pontén has found, Linneaus himself often criticised fashions of the period. When it came to hair, he was critical of the use of wigs, believing they weakened the skull. The weakened skull was then more exposed to cold temperatures. However, Linneaus still wore a wig himself, as befitting his profession and social status. The rationale was that since this had already weakened his skull, he had to continue to wear it to protect his head from the cold.[23]

To summarise, a certain level of care for one's appearance was expected, and fashions were inescapable even for the men of science who sometimes criticised them. Accepting this, Linneaus and his acolytes could disseminate knowledge about cosmetic hair dyes. As long as the remedies were derived from Swedish plants, this was in accordance with patriotic household ideology, even if they were detrimental to the health of the body.

Hair in eighteenth-century housekeeping manuals and medical texts

In the medical discourse of the period, haircare could also be defended as a way of maintaining cleanliness, neatness, and health. Certain hair treatments were sometimes provided in physicians' medical texts in the

21 Ibid., 'no. 21,' 27.

22 This description is found on the Swedish Natural history museum's website 'Den virtuella floran,' http://linnaeus.nrm.se/flora/di/lentibularia/pingu/pingvul.html. Accessed 24 June 2021.

23 Windahl Pontén, *Kiär hustru*, 179–180.

eighteenth century, even though they could be regarded as having a cosmetic function. Hair loss, for instance, was viewed both as a symptom of illness and as a medical problem on its own. As early as 1709, the physician and founder of Uppsala University hospital Lars Roberg translated a medical handbook containing, among other things, recipes for concoctions to treat hair loss, and to make hair grow thick. He recommended tinctures of liquorice and wormwood, as well as regularly cutting hair in order to get it to grow evenly.[24] In a book of household remedies aimed at people who had no access to doctors, first published in 1759, the Finnish physician Johan Haartman recommended combing and cutting hair regularly as a way to avoid hair loss.[25]

In a dissertation about scrofula, scabs, and sores from 1772, Pehr Bjerchén discussed how bumps and sores that children got on their heads could become infected if left untreated. The best way to forestall this was to keep children's heads clean through careful combing.[26] Rather than washing, combing was the recommended way to keep one's head clean in the eighteenth century. Such a recommendation was so widespread that in 1788, a writer in the journal *Stockholms-posten* joked about the 'science of hair combing.'[27] That academic physicians promoted this practice as a way to maintain healthy hair and a healthy scalp shows how it was indeed well established in the medical science of that time.

Recipe books anchored in practical housekeeping and folk remedies could include hair and skin treatments along with recipes for food and remedies for illnesses. In author and housekeeper Cajsa Warg's bestselling cookbook from 1755, a recipe for pomade was included. Its main ingredient was bacon grease. The preparation took sixteen days, and the amount would last a year according to Warg.[28] She did not state how or why it was used, but it was clearly a necessity for the household, given the amount of work to prepare it and that it was to be kept in stock. Making pomade was thus a part of 'housekeeping science,' according to Warg's definition, which she outlined in the book's introduction.[29] Pomades, popular throughout the eighteenth century, straddled the line between

24 Roberg, *Den barmhertige samariten*, 99.

25 No. 74, Swe. '*hårlopp*' in Haartman, *Tydelig Underrättelse*, 225. On Haartman, see also Charlotta Forss's chapter in this volume.

26 Bjerchén*Inträdes tal*, 29. On Bjerchén, see also Hjalmar Fors's chapter in this volume.

27 *Stockholms-posten*, 11 April 1788, 1. See also Åkerman, *Bepröfvade medel*, 10; Rowland (trans. Fågelberg), *Filosofisk och praktisk afhandling*, 17; Corson, *Fashions in Hair*, 266.

28 Warg, *Hjelpreda i Hushållningen*, 163.

29 Ibid., ii.

cosmetics and medicine. As beauty products, they promoted vanity, while as medical hair treatments they kept the scalp neat and clean, preserving health.[30]

Emma Marckiewicz has observed that in private handwritten books on housekeeping, the distinctions between food, beauty treatments, and health treatments were not rigidly fixed.[31] Cajsa Warg's cookbook contained not only recipes for food, but for cloth dyes and medicines to treat sick animals. Warg's cookbook thus resembled the private books on housekeeping Marckiewicz discusses, rather than latter-day cookbooks that focus exclusively on food. In Sweden, the influence of such housekeeping books continued in published literature well into the nineteenth century. *Allmän Hushålls-och Konstbok* (General household and artisanal handbook), translated by S. N. Wahrman and published in 1805, contained recipes for all sorts of things, including hair powder, pomades and hair dyes. *Handbok I Husmedicinen* (Handbook in Household Medicine), published in 1840 and intended to aid those who did not have access to doctors in a similar way to Haartman's book of medicines from 1759, contained a recipe to cure hair loss.[32]

It is established then that hair treatments could be found in the writings of renowned scientists of the period, and also in popular housekeeping books without formal scientific merits. As a matter of fact, there was no strong opposition to what would later be called folk medicine among medical practitioners, although charlatanism was criticised.[33] From a modern perspective, *En liten dock nyttig Örte-Bok* (A small but useful herb-book) can be classified as something closer to folk medicine than the publications of the scientists and physicians Roberg, Linneaus, Haartman, and Bjerchén.[34] This book was composed from a list of the medical uses of different herbs. It was first published in 1741 and thus predated Linneaus's and Aspelin's *Flora*. It continued to be reprinted until 1869. Unlike the *Flora Oeconomica*, it is unknown how *En liten dock nyttig Örte-Bok*'s information was collected, and the advice was eclectic. It recommended mugwort to both cure hair ailments, and at the same time, make hair grow long and beautiful.[35] It recommended sage as a way to

30 Brown, *Skönhetens mask*, 154.

31 Markiewicz, 'Hair, Wigs and Wig-Wearing,' 74 –75.

32 Wahrman, *Allmän Hushålls- och Konstbok*, 87–89, 181, 347; Wistrand, *Handbok i Husmedicinen*, 258.

33 Ling, *Kärringmedicin*, 64.

34 This is a reprinting from 1788. The original was printed in Strängnäs, 1741.

35 Swe. '*Gråbo*,' no. 130, 31.

strengthen one's memory, make hair grow, and dye it black.[36] In short, the book made little distinction between cures for physical ailments and cosmetic treatments.

In a similar vein, the companion books *Den sluga och förståndiga gubben* (The clever and sensible old man) from 1758 and *Den kloka och husaktiga gumman* (The wise and frugal old woman) from 1762 could be classed as examples of a commercialised folk medicine. As their titles show, they both presented the authors as old figures of tradition who possessed wisdom that separated them from the medical establishment of that time. Both books contained identical recipes to stimulate hair growth and treat baldness, advising readers to rub the scalp with combination of egg oil and a dried, pulverised frog.[37] In newspapers from the 1770s and 1780s, frogs were recommended as a cure to help people afflicted with scurvy on their scalps.[38] Frogs were associated with magic, and in folk remedies they could be used for many things. People continued to utilise them to stimulate hair growth in some regions of Sweden into the twentieth century.[39] If the use of frogs was connected to folklore however, eggs were more often associated with haircare as a beauty treatment, necessary to keep curls intact. Eggs frequently occurred as an ingredient in other cosmetic haircare recipes of the late eighteenth and early nineteenth century.[40]

Because they interlinked cosmetic hair treatments and medicinal treatments, the books examined here were precursors to a type of specialised literature on hair that would become available in Sweden in the nineteenth century once the powdered wig became unfashionable. It is possible that the loss of wigs created a need for more haircare for men belonging to the elite, the group that had used wigs the most. However, there was also a medicalised discourse surrounding the wig in the 1780s that might have contributed to the wig's decline in popularity.

36 Ibid. Swe. '*Salvia*,' no. 34, 12.

37 Bröms, *Den sluga och förståndiga gubben*, 164; Bruno, *Den kloka och husaktiga gumman*, 3.

38 *Stockholms Weckoblad*, 9 April 1774, 5; *Carlstads Weckotidningar*, 15 June 1781, 4.

39 Tillhagen, *Folklig läkekonst*, 266.

40 For other examples of hair treatments advising the use of egg, as a way to both curl it and stimulate hair growth, see Lindh, *Underrättelser för fruntimmer, I synnerhet hörande til toiletten* (*Information for young women, especially regarding the toilette*), 19, and *Konsten att blifwa Tio år yngre* (*The Art of becoming Ten years younger*), 66. In 1741, an anonymous author advised using eggs to treat scabs on children's heads in *Naturliga OECONOMIE och Hushålds Reglor, Samt Hus REMEDIA Eller Läkedomar, Som en försigtig håshållare* (*utan at söka apoteket*) *med stor nytta och ringa omkostnad säkert bruka kan* (*Natural Oeconomie and Household rules, and House Remedies or Medicines*), 19.

As mentioned, wigs were primarily a fashion for men in the late eighteenth century. While some women did wear wigs, it was more common for women to create elaborate hairstyles using their own long hair, often adding extensions.[41] This meant that the health concerns regarding wigs that were expressed in journals like *Stockholms-posten* targeted male vanity as a health hazard. A patriotic economic perspective dominated a series of critiques of men's hair fashions in *Stockholms-posten* in 1788. They linked the economic problems caused by elaborate hair fashions on a national level with the health problems individual fashion victims might suffer. In one of the pieces, the author argued that the work of creating wigs robbed the nation of labourers who belonged in sectors that Sweden's economic thinkers recognised as important: agriculture, mining, metal works, and handicrafts. In addition to this, wigs and elaborate hairstyles destroyed the health of their wearers:

> the strange fashion of the hair now separates a large amount of people from the State, and the coiffed must with sadness lose their time, their money, and with powder, pomade, scents and finally with the associated lack of a hat, their health.[42]

Not wearing a hat or a cap could produce a head cold, but an elaborate hairstyle meant people could not wear hats that covered the head fully, a reference to the perception that French fashions were ill-suited to the Nordic climate.

Another article on the same topic explored the health problems men in particular suffered through this fashion. Too much hair combing was to blame for 'now common' headaches.[43] Furthermore, powder, pomade and wigs blocked natural evaporations from the head. Scented powder caused skin irritations, and 'A long habit and constant use of odours makes him feeble, useless in all undertakings, and perhaps brings him to a premature death.'[44] The author characterised the use of wigs and hair treatments as a way for men to recapture their lost youth by imitating younger men.[45] This concern would recur in manuals for haircare published in the early nineteenth century.

41 Fawcett, 'Self and Society,' 40; Corson, *Fashions in Hair*, 261.

42 *Stockholms-posten*, 25 April 1788, 1.

43 *Stockholms-posten*, 11 April 1788, 3.

44 Ibid.

45 Ibid.

Hair treatments for men and women: gendering an emerging market in the nineteenth century.

A contrast to the diverse recipe collections of the previous century, recipe books exclusively for cosmetic treatments, including for hair, were published in Swedish in the first decade of the nineteenth century. These were Johan Pehr Lundström's *Underrättelser om Tillwerkningssättet af de finaste Fransyska och Italienska Twålsorter och Pomador* (Notifications on the preparation of the finest French and Italian soaps and Pomades) in 1807, and *Kallopistria, eller Toilett-konst för den eleganta verlden* (Kallopistria, or Toilette-art for the elegant world) attributed to the German pharmacist Johann Trommsdorff and translated to Swedish in 1808. In short introductions, the authors of these two works justified their focus on beauty treatments by linking their recipes to cultural practices from other nations such as France.[46] In the 1820s, another manual, *Konsten att blifva Tio år yngre* (The art of becoming ten years younger) was published. This manual combined recipes for hair and skin treatments with advice on exercise and dieting, making an explicit connection between exterior beauty and inner health.

Manuals specifically for hair treatments were also published in the first half of the nineteenth century. For one of these manuals, the original version is known and available: the Englishman Alexander Rowland's (1747–1823) *A Practical and Philosophical Treatise on the Human Hair.* The original was published in 1816, and Fredrik Louis Fågelberg's Swedish translation, *Filosofisk och Praktisk Afhandling angående Hufvudhåren,* was published in 1827. The same year, the orthopedic physician Nils Åkerman translated a book about preventing hair loss, called *Beprövade Medel att förekomma Hårets bortfallande* (Proven agents for preventing the loss of hair). Similar subjects were covered in the 1840s in Dr Francis Woolstone's *Om Hufvudets Kalhet* (On the baldness of the head), and in *Grundlig Anvisning till Bot för all slags Flintskallighet* (Thorough instruction to cures for all kinds of baldness), attributed to 'Dr U. Redelich.' Both books were published in 1842. The final section of this chapter focuses on the emergence of these manuals and what they meant for the further medicalisation of haircare in Swedish society and for the way hair was gendered.

The market for this type of literature was growing in this period. The publication of these books does not, however, mean that Swedish people had no access to manuals on haircare before 1827. The genre appeared earlier in countries like England and France. One example was the French physician

46 Lundström, *Underrättelser*, introduction; Söderström, *Kallopistria*, 2.

Pierre-Joseph Buc'Hoz's guide to cosmetics and haircare from 1771, *Toilette De Flore: Ou Essai Sur Les Plantes Et Les Fleurs Qui Peuvent Servir D'Ornement Aux Dames*. From 1772 and throughout the 1780s, advertisements in newspapers and journals show this guide was available in Stockholm and Gothenburg. From 1792 to at least 1816, an English translation was also available on the Swedish market.[47] The readership would have been restricted to an educated elite who read French or English, but knowledge of new fashions in haircare could still have spread to wider segments of society via these books. The earlier availability of these types of books in French and English certainly paved the way for Swedish manuals in the nineteenth century, demonstrating that a market existed for them.

The new manuals in Swedish reflected and commented on some of the changes in the hair fashions of this period, as well as changes in the market for products. Out of these authors, Francis Woolstone wrote the most extensively about wigs, mainly in a negative way. Woolstone was concerned about how heavy wigs prevented the head's healthy evaporations. He warned that a tight-set wig kept the head too warm, leading to blood congestions that could cause eye sickness, deafness, and strokes.[48] The similarities between Woolstone's concerns and those presented in *Stockholms-posten* and other journals in the 1780s gives an indication that the original version of this manual might have been published decades earlier than 1842. According to the cover, the Swedish version was a translation of the sixteenth edition of an English work. However, its translation and publication in 1842 is evidence that these ideas were still in circulation in Sweden at that time, regardless of when and where they had originated.

The translation of Alexander Rowland's book was published closer in time to its original edition and did not dwell as much on the dangers of wigs. Rowland had worked as a hairdresser himself, and the main purpose of his book was to promote Macassar oil, a hair oil he had invented using ingredients imported from the Dutch East Indies. Advertisements for Macassar oil appeared in various journals and newspapers in the southern, western, and eastern regions of Sweden. They began in 1825, two years prior to the book's translation, and continued to appear well into the 1830s.[49]

47 *Dagligt Allehanda*, 20 July 1772, 3; *Götheborgs Allehanda*, 27 March 1781, 4; *Hwad Nytt?*, 2 March 1781, 8; *Hwad Nytt?*, 12 November 1781, 8; *Götheborgs Tidningar*, 8 November 1787, 4; *Dagligt Allehanda*, 18 October 1787, 3. For advertisements for the English version, see *Dagligt Allehanda*, 24 January 1792, 9; *Dagligt Allehanda*, 23 April 1812, 6; *Dagligt Allehanda*, 5 October 1816, 5.

48 Woolstone, *Om hufvudets kalhet*, 10–12.

49 For examples of these advertisements, see: *Dagligt Allehanda*, 26 October 1825, 6; ibid., 29 October 1825, 6; *Lunds Weckoblad*, 8 October 1831, 4; *Hallands Läns Tidning*, 22 June 1837, 4;

The physician Nils Åkerman translated a book of cures for hair loss. He did not provide information about the original author the way Fågelberg had done, so this will be referred to as Åkerman's work. This book was published in 1827, the same year as Fågelberg's translation of Rowland. Åkerman made a reference to this work and its advertising campaign, stating that though Macassar oil was heavily promoted, it was in fact not the only useful treatment.[50] Åkerman instead included several recipes for treatments where the main ingredients, apart from scents, were 'pure, clean fat,' swine fat or beef fat, sometimes with an addition of white wax.[51] These recipes were not dissimilar to the one found in Cajsa Warg's cookbook from 1755. Cinchona bark was the only colonial product Åkerman recommended, and he advised that it should only be used in cases when people had cut their hair short and wanted to stimulate its growth.[52] The main topic of the book was hair loss due to illness, and for this his recipes used homegrown ingredients.

Åkerman's and Rowland's books both show the effects of the changing commercial market in Sweden, where products from Europe's colonies had become more available and were being heavily promoted as superior to previous solutions. However, Åkerman and Rowland presented competing visions. Rowland's book was concentrated on promoting a specific new product. With his homegrown ingredients and criticism of the promotion for Macassar oil, Åkerman was in some ways still writing in the tradition of medical handbooks of the eighteenth century. The writing was influenced by the ideals of the household economy and aimed towards a readership that might not have access to doctors and medicines provided in towns. Manuals like Rowland's and Åkerman's confirmed a market for hair products was growing in Sweden, but also that this market growth happened slowly, and that the reception of foreign hair products was not wholly positive.

When it came to the connection between hair and gender, there is a great deal of ambiguity regarding who the early cosmetic manuals and books' ideal readers were. This goes back to French and English precursors like *Toilette De Flore*. Despite its title and the introduction addressing 'dames,' the *Toilette De Flore* was not just meant for women readers; indeed,

Göteborgs Handels- och Sjöfartstidning, 8 August 1837, 2; *Wadstenabladet*, 10 November 1838, 4; *Skånska Posten*, 23 January 1839, 4; *Correspondenten*, 6 February 1839, 4; *Dagligt Allehanda*, 13 June 1839, 3; *Aftonbladet*, 7 August 1839, 6; *Östgöta Correspondenten*, 7 December 1839, 4. These are not all the adverts available, but provide evidence of the geographical scope of the campaign in Sweden.

50 Åkerman, *Bepröfvade medel*, 15.

51 Åkerman, *Bepröfvade medel*, 12–14.

52 Ibid., 15–16.

it contained a recipe for a beard dye.[53] None of the Swedish texts published before 1800, which are examined here, stated which gender should use their recipes. In the first decade of the nineteenth century, neither Moses Söderström's nor Johan Pehr Lundström's books on pomades revealed who should use them.

As mentioned, microscopic studies had shown that hair itself had no gender, though the body it came from did. In the seventeenth century, the idea that hair had no gender was not always accepted by the general population. In English Puritan tracts in the mid-1600s, wigs were criticised for transgressing gendered boundaries, since the wigs made of human hair certainly used hair collected from women.[54] In Sweden in 1695, the theologian and Vice-chancellor of Uppsala University Jesper Swedberg echoed this critique.[55] A similar concern was expressed in Francis Woolstone's book, published in Swedish more than a century later. According to Woolstone, the hairs of a wig often came either from fallen women, 'for a proper person would surely not want to sell their own hair,' or from hospital patients, making them contaminated with disease.[56] The fact that hair was both of the body and something that could be removed and transported to another body meant that hair could be interpreted in different, contradictory ways throughout the eighteenth and early nineteenth centuries.

One clearly gendered aspect of haircare was visible in the way the manuals were marketed. The idea that women were particularly concerned with beauty was visible in the advertising for the manuals, as well as in the introductory addresses. *Konsten att blifva Tio år yngre* was addressed to 'herrar och fruntimmer,' gentlemen and ladies, but despite this, its main focus seemed to be female readers. It contained two lengthy introductions that were addressed to women, one that discussed the requisites of female beauty according to men, and one that highlighted the benefits women reaped by exercising regularly.[57] This claim was similar to the arguments a number of prominent French physicians made for women's exercise regimes later, in the mid-nineteenth century. They stated that gaining beauty and grace rather than health and strength was the ultimate aim of women's exercise.[58] However, *Konsten att blifva Tio år yngre* did mention health as

53 Buc'hoz, English ed., *Toilet of the Flora* 1772, 'No. 18, To change the Hair or Beard Black,' 11. For recipes to prevent baldness, see also 'no. 9' and 'no. 11,' 8.

54 Festa, 'Personal Effects,' 49.

55 Möller, *Lyx och mode*, 9, 63.

56 Woolstone, *Om hufvudets kalhet*, 12–13.

57 Anonymous author, *Konsten*, 1–12, 13–19.

58 Stewart, *For Health and Beauty*, 154.

essential for women's beauty. Regular exercise was a way of achieving that.[59] Health and beauty were thus linked for women, but unlike in medical books and housekeeping books of the previous century, beauty was the main goal.

When it came to addressing men, the 'herrar' of the title, *Konsten att blifva Tio år yngre* added a note to a recipe for hair dyes saying they could also be used for sideburns and moustaches. This meant that, like *Toilette De Flore*, the book contained information relevant for both men and women, but its introductory chapters were exclusively concerned with women's beauty regimes.[60] When Fågelberg translated Alexander Rowland's book into Swedish in 1827, he also placed advertisements in journals that were addressed 'in particular, to the ladies who place a value on beautiful hair.'[61] However, in the first section of the text, he mentioned the ability of Rowland's hair oil to cure baldness, an affliction mostly suffered by men. In short, the subjects of interest for men in these books were toned down in the advertising as well as in their introductions, while feminine beauty was played up. The men's aims with haircare were thus not discussed in terms of beauty, but related to health.

In the books about curing hair loss, baldness was presented as a sign that a young man was aging too quickly. After a certain point, the books all stated that it was normal for a man to lose his hair, but not before the age of thirty or forty. This age limit varied from book to book. Hair loss was described as a matter of concern, and men should take measures to prevent it. Rowland stated that the body's fluids could change over time, and that this was apparent in a weakening of hair along with a weakening constitution.[62] The hair treatments offered in the books were a part of treating that weakness. One thing the books about baldness all contained was advice on diets and exercise to prevent hair loss. The health of the body was the ultimate cause of the hair's ailments because this affected the body's ability to produce the fluids necessary to protect the hair.[63]

Gender divisions were not completely rigid. Even when it came to baldness, the differences between male and female bodies were less distinct than presumed at first glance. Rowland, Åkerman, Woolstone, and Redelich all acknowledged that though men were more prone to going bald, certain ailments could also make women lose their hair, such as anxiety, illnesses

59 Anonymous author, *Konsten*, 14.

60 Ibid., 62.

61 *Wisby Weckoblad*, 3 March 1827, 4; *Helsingborgsposten*, 7 April 1827, 3.

62 Rowland (trans. Fågelberg), *Filosofisk och praktisk afhandling*, 6, 13.

63 Åkerman, *Bepröfvade medel*, 12; Rowland (trans. Fågelberg), *Filosofisk och praktisk afhandling*, 12; Redelich, *Grundlig anvisning*, 2, 9; Woolstone, *Om hufvudets kalhet*, 24.

or childbirth.[64] Redelich alleged that masturbation could make a person lose their hair because it caused the body to lose an excessive amount of semen. This would seem to target men, but even that is not entirely clear. Though the medical establishment had begun to reject them at that time, Redelich might still have ascribed to Aristotelian and Galenic theories claiming that women, as well as men, produced semen. These theories continued to occur in popular scientific literature even in the 1840s.[65] Hair generally grew in different ways and places according to gender, a fact that was frequently explained with humoral theories, but, it also had transgressive qualities.[66] The haircare manuals of the nineteenth century claimed hair could be managed and altered with the proper treatments, regardless of what gender and balance of humours the body might originally possess. However, though hair was not exclusively connected to gender, there was nevertheless a strong tendency towards gendering descriptions of hair and haircare more in the haircare manuals and advertising in the early nineteenth century when compared to the medical textbooks and housekeeping books of the eighteenth century.

Conclusion

This chapter concludes with some observations on how and why haircare was gendered in Sweden in the late eighteenth and early nineteenth centuries, and how this correlated with a shifting understanding of health. It was clear that hair afflictions could affect different genders to different extents, but hair itself did not have to be a gendered material. From an economic standpoint, this meant that in the nineteenth century, cosmetic manuals could simultaneously market themselves to both genders. As some of the examples discussed above have shown, these manuals did so in different ways. In the first decades of the nineteenth century, there emerged a difference in the way the manuals were addressed to men and women. Hair was identified as a facet of beauty when it came to women, whereas when the address was to men, the medical aspect of haircare was promoted. Cosmetic hair dyes for men, with no apparent health benefits, were hidden within

64 Rowland (trans. Fågelberg), *Filosofisk och praktisk afhandling*, 10; Redelich, *Grundlig anvisning*, 15; Woolstone, *Om hufvudets kalhet*, 22.
65 Redelich, *Grundlig anvisning*, 17–20; Hitchcock, *English Sexualities*, 43, 46; Laqueur, *Making Sex*, 56, 66.
66 Markiewicz, 'Hair, Wigs and Wig-Wearing,' 52, 57.

books whose introductions mainly addressed female readers. This difference in address had been less apparent in the eighteenth century, when haircare recipes were the providence of housekeeping books and medical texts.

Regardless of the transgressive power of hair, the debates about men's hairstyles in *Stockholm-posten* in 1788 showed that haircare and wig-wearing mainly were men's habits, and men's problems. They connected the excessive use of wigs and hair products to ill health and concerns with aging. In using artificial methods, men tried to prevent their aging, but instead these methods caused them to age more rapidly, and with less dignity. Nineteenth-century literature on hair in Sweden continued to connect haircare to men's fear of aging. With some exceptions, these manuals can be assumed to have had a wider male than female readership because of their focus on curing baldness, a more common affliction for men. The books all connected the health of the hair to the health of the body, describing healthy hair as an aspect of healthy youth, and promoting diets and exercise. Even books mainly written to sell particular treatments, like Alexander Rowland's *Filosofisk och praktisk afhandling angående hufvudhåren*, acknowledged that the qualities of hair were connected to the body it came from, thus reiterating humoral theories.

A broad comparison between the different forms of literature presented here reveals that, in Puritan tracts of the late seventeenth century, hair was presumed to have innate qualities associated with the body it came from. However, the market for wigs and recipe books for medicines and cosmetics expanded in the 1700s. In eighteenth-century medical books and housekeeping books, the innately gendered qualities of hair were toned down. If any of the texts from that time had moral objections to haircare and wigs, they dealt more with the economic problems that vanity and the consumption of foreign goods caused the nation. They also focused on the health problems these practices were presumed to cause, for men in particular. In nineteenth-century recipe books for haircare, there would seem to have been a commercial interest for those selling new recipes and products to regard hair as something that could be altered, rather than as an intrinsic part of the body. This was also what both microscopic studies of hair and the widespread use of wigs in the previous century had seemed to indicate. That meant that hair could be commodified, and that its quality could be affected by dyes, medicines, and products, rather than being defined by the body it came from. However, the growth of a market for men's haircare that was promoted by physicians like Nils Åkerman and translators like Fredrik Louis Fågelberg, and the emergence of advertisements for products targeted at men and treatments in journals and newspapers, reveal a change from the eighteenth century. In the haircare discourse related to men, the hair used in wigs was characterised as weakening, disease-creating, and fake. On the other hand, a full head of natural hair resulted from a combination of treatments, certain diets, and exercise, and was a signifier of health and vitality. In this way, hair became reattached to the body in the nineteenth century, and it also became more gendered than it had been in the 1700s.

Bibliography

Printed works

Aftonbladet, 7 August 1839.

Anonymous. *Konsten att blifva tio år yngre. En handbok för herrar och fruntimmer, som vilja förhöja, bibehålla eller återställa sin ungdomsskönhet. Innehållande 100:de fullt godkända recepter till förskönande af alla kroppens delar, i synnerhet: ansigtet, bröstet, händerna, håret, ögonen, tänderna etc., jemte medel att reparera deras bristfälligheter samt conservera dem till ålderdomen.* Stockholm: Elméns & Granbergs tryckeri, 1828.

Anonymous. *Kårt och redig Underwisning om Färge-Konsten, Som lärer, At sätta allehanda färgor på Siden – Ylle – och Linne – Tygern, Jämte en liten Tilökning Om åtskilliga färgor på hår, Det Allmänna Bästa til tjenst och nytta ifrån Ängelskan öfwersatt*). Stockholm: Lars Salvius, 1747.

Anonymous. *En liten dock nyttig örte-bok, hwar utinnan mästadelen af wåre inhemske trä och gräs til sine dygder emot åtskillige sjukdomar warda beskrefne. Efter mångens åstundan och trägna begäran å nyo uplagde. Linköping, Fredrich Schonberg: och Björkegrens änka 1788.* Linköping, 1788.

Aspelin, Elias. *Flora oeconomica eller Hushållsnyttan af de i Sverige wildt wäxande örter, under Carl Linnaei inseende uti et academiskt prof, år 1748 på latin och nu på modersmålet utgifwen av Elias Aspelin.* Uppsala, 1748.

Åkerman, Nils. *Bepröfvade medel att förekomma hårets bortfallande, befordra hårvexten, och åstadkomma att äfven kala ställen på hufvudet åter betäckas af hår. Öfversättning.* Stockholm: Marquardska boktryckeriet, 1827.

Bjerchén, Pehr. *Inträdes tal om kräftskadors, scrophulöse och veneriske sårs och svullnaders igenkännande. Hållit för kongl. collegium medicum, den 18 October 1771, af Pehr Bierchén ... På kongl. collegii befallning.* Stockholm, 1772.

Bruno, Georg Fredrik. *Den kloka och husaktiga gumman, hwilken, igenom egen och andras förfarenhet, uptäcker hwarjehanda nyttiga och nödiga hus-curer, så wäl för människor som kreatur, jämte hwad eljest nödwändigt och nyttigt pröfwas at weta, uti et hushåll så i städerna, som på landet.* Stockholm, 1762.

Bröms, Pehr. *Den sluga och förståndiga gubben, som lärer de oförfarna både i städerna och på landet, at igenom hwarjehanda hus-curer, hela och bota mångfaldiga sjukdomar, så wäl hos människor, som fänad; jämte mycket annat, som kan tjäna til förmon och nytta i åtskilliga hushålls-stycken.* Stockholm, 1757.

Buc'hoz, Pierre-Joseph (English translation). *The toilet of Flora; or, a collection of the most simple and approved methods of preparing baths, essences, pomatums, ... With receipts for cosmetics of every kind, ... For the use of the ladies. Improved from the French of M. Buchoz, M.D.* London: J. Murray and W. Nicoll, 1772.

Carlstads Weckotidningar, 15 June 1781.

Correspondenten, 6 February 1839.

Dagligt Allehanda, 20 July 1772.

Dagligt Allehanda, 18 October 1787.

Dagligt Allehanda, 24 January 1792.

Dagligt Allehanda, 23 April 1812.

Dagligt Allehanda, 5 October 1816.

Dagligt Allehanda, 16 October 1825.

Dagligt Allehanda, 13 June 1839.

Göteborgs Handels- och Sjöfartstidning, 8 August 1837.

Götheborgs Allehanda, 27 March 1781.

Götheborgs Tidningar, 8 November 1787.

Haartman, Johan. *Tydelig underrättelse, om de mäst gångbara sjukdomars kännande och motande, genom lätta och enfalliga hus-medel; samt et litet res- och hus-apothek; dem til tjenst, som ej hafwa tilfälle at rådfråga läkare, med åtskilliga förbätringar: och tilökningar, andra gången sammanfattad och utgifwen af Joh. Joh:son Haartman ... Åbo, tryckt hos Joh. Christoph. Frenckell, 1765.* Uppsala, 1963.

Hallands Läns Tidning, 2 June 1837.

Helsingborgsposten, 7 April 1827.

Hoffman, Nicolaus Ingewald. *Naturliga OECONOMIE och Hushålds Reglor, Samt Hus REMEDIA Eller Läkedomar, Som en försigtig håshållare (utan at söka apoteket) med stor nytta och ringa omkostnad säkert bruka kan.* Stockholm 1741.

Hwad Nytt?, 3 March 1781.

Hwad Nytt?, 12 November 1781.

Lindh, Johan Pehr. *Underrättelser för fruntimmer, I synnerhet hörande til toiletten.* Stockholm, [unknown date, 1790s].

Lunds Weckoblad, 10 August 1831.

Lundström, Johan Pehr. *Underrättelser om tillverkningssättet af de finaste fransyska och italienska twålsorter och pomador m.m.: Saml. och utg.* Jönköping, 1807.

Post- och inrikes Tidningar, 23 January 1772.

Redelich, U. *Grundlig anvisning till Bot för all slags Flintskallighet som icke beror af en hög ålder. För Läkare och Icke-läkare. Af Dr U. Redelich.* Gävle: A. P. Landin, 1842.

Roberg, Lars. *Den barmhertige samariten det är Wälmeent rådh och underrättelse, huruledes man allahanda menniskians in- och utwärtes siukdommar och bräcklighet medh ringa, oanseenlige, doch godfundne läkedommar hielpa skall, den fattigom och särdeles på landet boendom till nytta och gagn beskrifwit. Af Elias Beynon den yngre. Samt och ett kort uttåg aff Johan Guffers lillas Huuszapoteek af samma innehåld. Stockholm, tryckt hoos Julius G. Matthiæ åhr 1709.* Stockholm, 1709

Rowland, Alexander (translated by Fredrik Louis Fågelberg). *Filosofisk och praktisk afhandling angående hufvudhåren, jemte en beskrifning om deras växt och position, de sjukdomar för hvilka de äro föremål, och medel som kunna hindra och bota dem; samt underrättelse för föräldrar rörande deras : barns hår, jemte en beskrifning om macassar-hår-oljans ojemförliga egenskaper; utgifven till de personer som sätta värde på vackert hår, af Rowland ... elev af Joshon Brook ... Öfversatt från franskan af F.L. Fågelberg.* Wisby: Ax. Cedergren, 1827.

Skånska Posten, 23 January 1839.

Stockholm magistrate. 'Publication Angående Bönhaseri Uti Peruque-makare Ämbetet. Stockholms Rådhus den 7. December A:o 1733.' Stockholm, 7 December 1733.

Stockholm magistrate. 'Ytterligare Kungörelse Och Förbud emot Bönhaseri uti det Peruque-Makare Ämbetet tilhörande arbete. Gifwen Stockholms Rådhus den 17. December. År 1748.' Stockholm, 17 December 1748.

Stockholm magistrate. 'Kungörelse, at ej någon må med Hårs friserande och kammande eller Peruquers förfärdigande och säljande, Peruque-Makare-Ämbetet uti dess Handtwärk och näring förfördela. Gifwen Stockholms Rådhus den 17 juni1757.' Stockholm: Lars Salvius, 17 June 1757.

Stockholms-posten, 11 April 1788.

Stockholms-posten, 25 April 1788.

Stockholms Weckoblad, 9 April 1774.

Söderström, Moses. *Kallopistria, eller Toilett-konst för den eleganta verlden. En anledning att förfärdiga oskadliga parfymer och skönhetsmedel, pulver, pomador, smink, tvål, aromatiska bad och flera andra medel tjenliga att förhöja, bevara eller återställa: skönheten. Af d:r J. Barth. Trommsdorff ... Öfversatt af M. Söderström.* Stockholm, 1808.

Wadstenabladet, 10 November 1838.

Wahrman, Sven Niclas. *Allmän hushålls- och konstbok, eller Samling af utwalda föreskrifter til hushållares, handtwerkares, konstnärers och konstälskares tjenst af C.A.F. Hochheimer. ... Öfwersatt i sammandrag från tredje tyska upplagan af S. N. Wahrman, Första delen.* Örebro: Nils Magnus Lindh, 1805.

Warg, Cajsa. *Hjelpreda i hushållningen för unga fruentimber*, Stockholm: Lor. Ludv. Grefing, 1755.

Wisby Weckoblad, 3 March 1827.

Wistrand, August. *Handbok i husmedicinen : eller anwisning för igenkännandet och den enklaste behandlingen af inre och yttre sjukdomar, jemte en kort sundhetslära och wägledning för de wanligaste medikamenternas rätta bruk ... af A. Timoleon Wistrand ; genomsedd samt med ändringar och tillägg försedd af A. Hilarion Wistrand.* Stockholm, 1840.
Woolstone, Francis. *Om hufvudets kalhet eller anvisning att, på de ställen, der håret affallit, åstadkomma den vackraste och tätaste hårvext, jemte föreskrifter och försigtighetsmått vid nyttjandet af peruker och till förekommande af hårets affallande och grånande, samt grånadt hårs återställande till dess fordna färg.* Stockholm: L. J. Hjerta, 1842.
Östgöta Correspondenten, 7 December 1839.

Literature

Ågren, Maria. 'Introduction: Making a Living, Making a Difference.' In *Making a Living, Making a Difference: Gender and Work in Early Modern European Society*, edited by Maria Ågren, 1–23. New York: Oxford University Press, 2017.
Brown, Carolina. *Skönhetens Mask: Historia om Kropp och själv, ideal och verklighet.* Stockholm: Carlsson, 2011.
Corson, Richard. *Fashions in Hair: The First Five Thousand Years.* London: Peter Owens, 1965.
Earle, Rebecca. *Feeding the People: The Politics of the Potato.* Cambridge: Cambridge University Press, 2020.
Fawcett, Julia H. 'Self and Society: Women Wearing Wigs: A Short History of a Long Eighteenth-Century Problem.' In *A Cultural History of Hair in the Age of Enlightenment,* edited by Margaret K. Powell and Joseph Roach, 39–52. London: Bloomsbury Academic, 2019.
Festa, Lynn M. 'Personal Effects: Wigs and Possessive Individualism in the Long Eighteenth Century.' *Eighteenth-Century Life* 29, no. 2 (2005): 47–90.
Frängsmyr, Tore. 'Den gudomliga ekonomin: Religion och hushållning i 1700-talets Sverige.' *Lychnos 1971–1972* (1973): 217–243.
Grant, Mark. 'Steiner and the Humours: the Survival of Ancient Greek Science.' *British Journal of Educational Studies* 47, no. 1 (1999): 56–70.
Harvey, Karen. *The Little Republic: Masculinity and Domestic Authority in Eighteenth Century Britain.* Oxford: Oxford University Press, 2012.
Hitchcock, Tim. *English Sexualities, 1700–1800.* London: MacMillan, 1997.
Kwass, Michael. 'Big Hair: A Wig History of Consumption in Eighteenth-Century France.' *The American Historical Review* 111, no. 3 (2006): 631–659.
La Mettrie, Julien Offray de. *Machine Man and Other Writings*, edited by Ann Thomson. Cambridge: Cambridge University Press, 1996.

Laqueur, Thomas. *Making Sex: Body and Gender from the Greeks to Freud*. Cambridge, MA: Harvard University Press, 1990.

Laver, James. *Costume and Fashion: A Concise History*. London: Thames & Hudson, [1969] 1992.

Lindberg, Bo. *Praemia et poenae: Etik och straffrätt i Sverige i tidig ny tid*. Vol. 1, *Rättsordningen*. Uppsala: Uppsala universitet, 1992.

Lindström, Dag, Rosemarie Fiebranz, Jonas Lindström, Jan Mispelaere, and Göran Rydén. 'Working Together.' In *Making a Living, Making a Difference: Gender and Work in Early Modern European Society*, edited by Maria Ågren, 57–79. New York: Oxford University Press, 2017.

Lindström, Jonas, and Karin Hassan Jansson. 'Pigan i fadersväldet. Regler, undantag och mikrohistoriska möjligheter.' In *Historisk tidskrift* 137, no. 3 (2017): 351–378.

Ling, Sofia. *Kärringmedicin och vetenskap: Läkare och kvacksalverianklagade i Sverige omkring 1770–1870* (Old wives' Remedies and Science: Physicians and So-Called Quacks in Sweden, 1770 to 1870). Uppsala: Acta Universitatis Upsaliensis, 2004.

Markiewicz, Emma. 'Hair, Wigs and Wig Wearing in Eighteenth-Century England.' PhD diss., Warwick University, 2014. http://webcat.warwick.ac.uk/record=b2753822~S1.

Möller, Håkan. *Lyx och mode i stormaktstidens Sverige: Jesper Swedberg och kampen mot perukerna*. Stockholm: Atlantis, 2014.

Oldstone-Moore, Christopher. *Of Beards and Men: The Revealing History of Facial Hair*. Chicago: University of Chicago Press, 2015.

Powell, Manushag N. 'Class and Social Status: Hair and Social Boundaries.' In *A Cultural History of Hair in the Age of Enlightenment*, edited by Margaret K. Powell and Joseph Roach, 155–170. London: Bloomsbury Academic, 2019.

Powell, Margaret K., and Joseph Roach. 'Health and Hygiene.' In *A Cultural History of Hair in the Age of Enlightenment*, edited by Margaret K. Powell and Joseph Roach, 91–108. London: Bloomsbury Academic, 2019.

Rosenthal, Angela. 'Raising Hair.' *Eighteenth-Century Studies* 38, no. 1, 'Hair' (2004): 1–16.

Runefelt, Leif. *Dygden som välståndets grund: Dygd, nytta och egennytta i frihetstidens ekonomiska tänkande*. Stockholm: Stockholms universitet, 2005.

Runefelt, Leif. *Att hasta mot undergången: Anspråk, flyktighet, förställning i debatten om konsumtion i Sverige 1730–1830*. Lund: Nordic Academic Press, 2015.

Runefelt, Leif. *Hushållningens dygder: Affektlära, hushållningslära och ekonomiskt tänkande under svensk stormaktstid*. Stockholm: Almqvist & Wiksell International, 2001.

Singer, P. N. *Galen: Selected Works: Translated with an Introduction and Notes*. World's Classics. Oxford and New York: Oxford University Press, 1997.

Snook, Edith. 'Beautiful Hair, Health, and Privilege in Early Modern England.' *Journal for Early Modern Cultural Studies* 15, no. 4 (Fall 2015): 22–51.
Stewart, Mary Lynn. *For Health and Beauty. Physical Culture for French Women 1880s–1930s*. Baltimore and London: John Hopkins University Press, 2001.
Thomson, Ann. 'Animals, Humans, Machines and Thinking Matter, 1690–1707.' *Early Science and Medicine* 15, nos. 1–2 (2010): 3–37.
Tillhagen, Carl-Herman. *Folklig läkekonst*. 2nd ed. Stockholm: Hæggström, 1962.
Vermeulen, Heather V. 'Race and Ethnicity: Mortal Coils and Hair-Raising Revolutions: Styling "Race" in the Age of Enlightenment.' In *A Cultural History of Hair in the Age of Enlightenment,* edited by Margaret K. Powell and Joseph Roach, 135–154. London: Bloomsbury Academic, 2019.
Windahl Pontén, Annika. *Kiär hustru, wackra barn, bodde i ett palais: Identitet och materialitet i hushållet von Linné*. Uppsala: Acta Universitatis Upsaliensis, 2020.
Wright, John P. 'Metaphysics and Physiology: Mind, Body, and the Animal Economy in Eighteenth-Century Scotland.' In *Studies in the Philosophy of the Scottish Enlightenment,* edited by M. A. Stewart, 251–301. Oxford: Clarendon Press, 1990.

About the Author

Hedvig Widmalm is a Postdoctoral Researcher at Umeå University. Her research concerns economic doctrines and policies in early modern Sweden, with a focus on how norms and regulations influenced women's work in the eighteenth century.

9. Gender Norms and Early Modern Healthcare: Barber-Surgeons in Sweden c. 1600–1900

Maria Sjöberg

Abstract
In this article, gender coding will be analysed from a long-term perspective, c. 1600–1900. By following barber-surgeons, a male-coded and guild-based occupation, from 1600 to 1900, it is possible to infer what the gender norms were and how they changed. In Sweden, it seems clear that the regulations of the guild, on a formal level, included everyone in the household of the barber-surgeon; if necessary, the wife could take over her husband's business. This changed over time. At the end of the nineteenth century, it became formally permitted for women to train as barber-surgeons in their own right. Consequently, a long-term perspective reveals that preconceived notions concerning gender order have varied throughout history.

Keywords: gender, early modern, healthcare, barber-surgeon

Health and healthcare in the past

The World Health Organisation's 1946 definition of health, often referred to as fundamental in modern societies, embraces 'a state of complete physical, mental and social well-being, and not merely the absence of disease and infirmity.'[1] This definition is vague. Exactly what should be included in these three named aspects and with which strategies health is to be achieved can be widely discussed. The point here, however, is that the definition includes more than just the absence of disease. Irrespective of the debate surrounding how the definition should be perceived or practised, it is clear

1 *Läkartidningen*, 'Debate post.'

Eyice, M. and C. Forss (eds.), *Health and Society in Early Modern Sweden*.
Taylor & Francis Group 2024
DOI 10.5117/9789463724296_CH09

that, since the 1940s, concepts of health emphasise the experience of health conditions. This view proclaims a distinct shift in thoughts and attitudes, from a perspective in which disease and illness were natural parts of human life, as was the case in early modern times, towards a perspective in which the normal human condition is the absence of disease.[2] In earlier periods, the overall responsibility for a subject's health was obscure, and the possible measures to ensure health are at best a matter of relief and remedy. In more recent times, health has become a governmental responsibility with attempts for treatment improvements as well as preventive measures. This shift can also be illuminated linguistically. In the Swedish language of the sixteenth century, the concept of health alludes primarily to material welfare and prosperity – something desirable but almost completely dependent on God's will. In the early modern era, disease and poverty were inextricably linked. Not until later did the notion of health become separated from poverty and more explicitly associated with the body's useful functioning.[3]

Apart from living a godly life, there were few possibilities for human beings to secure their future health. The medical care provided at the time was focused on healing injuries and illnesses, not on preventing future ones. In the Ancient Nordic fairytale literature, the Icelandic sagas, it is well established that this kind of medical practice was performed by both women and men.[4] However, this changed over time, and healing gradually became formalised as a male activity. In that sense, various categories of healers and physicians underwent masculinisation. In current research, Christianity is considered to have caused this change in medical practice during the Middle Ages.[5] However, it is important to keep in mind that this process took place only on a formal level and seems to have been almost completed on an officially authorised level in the seventeenth century. However, the extent to which the household or family was involved in the concrete work with healthcare is unclear. Certainly, official healthcare practitioners were mostly men. On the other hand, as we will see in this chapter, in the legislation and the associated privileges, the emphasis on the importance of the household, including women, complicates the picture of the craft's gradual masculinisation process.

On the surface, barbers, barber-surgeons, doctors, bathers, and pharmacists were all male-coded and guild-based occupations, in contrast

2 The definition is of course most relevant for Western Europe.
3 *Svenska Akademiens Ordbok* (*SAOB*): 'hälsa,' 'välfärd,' 'välgång.'
4 Bergqvist, *Läkare och läkande*, 194–195.
5 Crawford, 'The Nadir of Western Medicine?,' 41–51.

to both the medieval and contemporary eras, when both genders could formally practise healthcare. In the late 1800s, practice changed again. Women became formally qualified as barber-surgeons and medical doctors, and nursing became a purely female profession. The gender pattern changed yet again in the twentieth century. The first male nurses qualified for certification in the 1950s and the first male midwives in the 1960s. Today in Sweden, the majority of doctors, nurses, and assistant nurses are women in both the private and public healthcare sectors. What caused this gender pattern shift to undergo such dramatic changes? An explanatory context must reasonably be linked to these changing gender norms in society, which is the central theme of this chapter.

In the following discussion, gender coding will be analysed from a long-term perspective, c. 1600–1900, focusing on women's formal practice of healthcare, particularly as barbers or barber-surgeons in Sweden. The fluctuations in gender coding will be specifically clarified through this occupation, from when it was a guild-based craft in the sixteenth century to when it became the responsibility of the military for specifically military healthcare during the seventeenth and eighteenth centuries. Later, during the nineteenth century, the occupation was almost divided into two branches. One gradually focused on surgery, which became a prestigious medical speciality, while the other retained the craft that initially justified the guild's privileges. The latter form of the occupation was also open to women. By following the history of barber-surgeons over the centuries, from 1600 to 1900, it should reasonably be possible to infer what the gender norms were during this period, and how they changed. At the same time, a long-term perspective brings with it certain challenges. Words and terms change meaning over time, and disease patterns vary occasionally, partly depending upon social conditions. Thus, the time-specific context runs the risk of being lost. On the other hand, a long-term perspective supports the fact that preconceived notions concerning the gender order have varied throughout history and can therefore change again. It is also clear that structural changes, often described as gender-neutral, have in fact been gendered. Hence, the purpose of this chapter is to analyse these value-bearing facts.

On the surface: a gradual masculinisation

Despite the dominant presence of Christianity and the growth of the church organisation, the heterogeneous collection of designations stating the kind of curative treatment offered by both women and men for payment remained the same for a long time. Designations like cupping, blood-letting, and bathing continued. Treatment methods and female healers are mentioned in folklore records.[6] In historical research, their presence is made visible in connection with legal interventions.[7] In short, Christianity, in relation to the emergence of the clergy, may have affected the opportunities for women to practise healthcare on a formal level. However, women involved in healthcare did not completely cease to exist, although they disappeared from formal positions. In the early modern era, another wave of masculinisation occurred, which was connected with the growing numbers of scientifically and formally educated doctors. This happened all over Europe, parallel to the organisation of licensed male healthcare practitioners into guilds and colleges in European cities.[8] At the same time, the legislation in several countries tried to enforce the abolishment of female healers.[9] In Sweden, medically orientated crafts such as barbers and bathers were organised as guilds. These guilds were mainly linked to Stockholm, while formally educated medical doctors were linked to both the faculty of medicine in Uppsala and, from 1663, to the Collegium Medicum in Stockholm.[10] Later, in 1778, pharmacists organised themselves into a society. Pharmacies, located in several cities, provided physicians and others with remedies. Moreover, all the parishes in Sweden were led by a clergyman who also practised healthcare.

Guilds, colleges, faculties, and the church were all male organisations and female healers were thus structurally excluded. Barbers in Sweden were recruited to the military first and foremost in the seventeenth and eighteenth centuries and these positions were not available to women. However, apart from that, healthcare organisation remained diversified with regard to gender.

The Reformation was unequivocally a factor in the diversification of healthcare in Sweden in the sixteenth century. After the dissolution of the monasteries, there was no obvious single institution that provided medical care, although the church continued to be formally responsible for healthcare

6 Tillhagen, *Folklig läkekonst*.

7 Oja, *Varken Gud eller natur*, 167; Jütte, *Ärzte, Heiler und Patienten*, 124–125; Runesson, *Blod, kött och tårar*, 94–96.

8 Guild formation and gradual masculinisation was a general trend in several occupations. See Merry E. Wiesner, 'Guilds, Male Bonding and Women's Work,' 125, 131; Lindström, *Skrå, stad, stat*, 84.

9 Radford Ruether, *Women and Redemption*, 115; Whaley, *Women and the Practice*, 26–47.

10 See also Hjalmar Fors's chapter in this volume.

and caring for the poor. This opened new opportunities for different groups to market their skills. In the 'grand narrative' of medical history, early modern healthcare is thus treated as very deficient. Those were good times for all kinds of charlatans, writes the Swedish historian Sten Lindroth.[11] With the gradual establishment of formally trained doctors of medicine in the seventeenth century, who could diagnose and treat illnesses on a scientific basis, practitioners of medical science began to compete against other groups who claimed to cure diseases. Thus, a main theme in the 'grand narrative' of medical history is how formally trained medical doctors competed against other practitioners of medicine and were finally victorious.[12]

A silent and perhaps unconscious point of departure in this 'success story' is that medicine, as practised by formally educated doctors in the seventeenth century, was based on the same kind of science as it is today. That opinion can be backed up by examining the medical books written by doctors of medicine during the seventeenth and eighteenth centuries. In 1686, Collegium Medicum published Sweden's first pharmacopoeia, *Pharmacopoeia Holmiensis: Galeno-chymica*, probably compiled by the doctors Johannes Ziervogel, Lars Roberg, and Urban Hjärne. All three were highly respected doctors and scholars in their time. Medicinal preparations included, for example, fats from humans, feral cats, dogs, and snakes, to mention but a few sources. Also included in these medicinal preparations for cures were human bones, mummy flesh, the brain bowls of hanged or beheaded people, moss from old skulls, and many other similar objects. The pharmacopoeia describes which diseases could be cured with the aid of the preparations mentioned, as well as the amounts, dimensions, and weights required. All of these were remedies that were rooted in a magical and religious world. The above-mentioned pharmacopoeia was not replaced with a new one until 1775 and illustrates the blurred boundaries between medicine as science and medicine as healing.[13]

Through the publication of detailed instructions, medical knowledge and accepted medical treatments were made available to literate people. Was this perhaps a time when, to a greater extent than before, medicine turned into folk medicine? Whatever the answer to that question, the published pharmacopoeia nevertheless emphasises that medical science and the medically trained doctors in the second half of the seventeenth century

11 Lindroth, *Svensk lärdomshistoria. Frihetstiden*, 414.

12 Lindroth, *Svensk lärdomshistoria. Frihetstiden*, 414; Brieger, 'History of Medicine'; Johannisson, *Medicinens öga*, 13–14.

13 Tillhagen, *Folklig läkekonst*, 14–15.

provided almost the same medical cures as other healthcare practitioners. Since then, however, the differences have become ever greater. But this development has been a slow process, perhaps due to the fact that formally educated medical doctors were mainly theoretically orientated, and to a lesser extent involved in actually practising healthcare.

Swedish historical research on medicine and healthcare has focused on conditions in the nineteenth and twentieth centuries, and that focus is on the emergence of science and the publicly funded healthcare organisation.[14] With a few important exceptions, Swedish historians have not studied in detail the practices of physicians without formal medical training, including barbers, in early modern times. Among these exceptions is the archaeologist Johanna Bergqvist's study on the professionalisation process in healing during the Middle Ages and the Renaissance. Her study covers a long period, 1100 to 1600, and examines perceptions of disease, affliction and injury, practitioners of the arts of healing, and finally, the various types of healing. Bergqvist argues that the Black Death and the following epidemics devastated domestic traditions of knowledge in the arts of healing. These circumstances forced a reorientation towards foreign medical education.[15] Her study provides background and context for this chapter's discussion. Bergqvist notes that several barber-surgeons were recruited from abroad, especially during the seventeenth-century wars, and for a long time it was not possible to acquire a formal medical degree in Sweden. Another source is Bo S. Lindberg, who has a background as a medically trained physician himself. He has studied the history of surgeons from the Middle Ages until the end of the nineteenth century. His focus is primarily on the formation of a profession, how individuals organised themselves, how they were trained and how they competed against doctors with formal medical training.[16] His study treats several aspects that are important for this chapter as well. A third source is Sofia Ling's study on old wives' remedies, and how science offers perspectives on the relationship between licensed and unlicensed healers that are useful for understanding the change in gender norms at the end of nineteenth century.[17] In addition to the sources mentioned above, there are several studies in which various types of healing are dealt with,

14 For example, Qvarsell, *Vårdens idéhistoria*; Qvarsell and Sundin, 'The Social and Cultural History of Medicine and Health in Sweden'; Berge, *Sjukvårdens underklass*; Johannisson, Nilsson, and Qvarsell, *Medicinen blir till vetenskap*.

15 Bergqvist, *Läkare och läkande*, 342–343.

16 Lindberg, *Kirurgernas historia*.

17 Ling, *Kärringmedicin och vetenskap*.

but not from the perspective of studying healthcare practice in the early modern era.

If the sparse Swedish historical research on this topic from an early modern perspective is viewed in an international context, the contrast is obvious. International research on the healthcare of older times has for several decades been both extensive and diverse. Practitioners of medicine and their experience-based knowledge as well as patients' perspectives have been investigated – with an emphasis on British contexts and conditions.[18] Certainly, there are attempts to diachronically analyse health, healthcare, responsibility, and medical thinking in the Nordic countries.[19] However, this research, on the medical science that eventually came to dominate other kinds of medicine, and which was already in ancient times documented in theoretical and philosophical writings, also indicates a bias in the research framework.[20] Experience-based medicine, practised by groups other than doctors with formal medical training, was based on practical skills that left their mark on written sources to a much lesser extent. Although the state of historical research in this field is now different from that of the 1970s, when the influential historian Sten Lindroth published his work on the history of ideas from the Middle Ages up to modernity, the practice of healthcare in the seventeenth and eighteenth centuries is still scarcely explored, partly due to the fact that the sources are only preserved in fragments.[21] This assessment applies not least to the role in healthcare of the barber, whose significance in Swedish medical history has most recently been investigated by the above-mentioned Bo S. Lindberg.

Barbers as a guild based on household organisation

The Swedish language provides three overlapping terms for barbers. Firstly, there was the 'bardskärare' (Ger. *bartschneider*), whose task was primarily to cut hair and shave beards, although they also practised simpler wound

18 The field of research is enormous, and just a few books are mentioned here. An overview of the historiography up to 1980 is given by Brieger, 'History of Medicine'; for an emphasis on practice, see Porter, *Patients and Practitioners*, *Health for Sale*, and *Cambridge History of Medicine*; for ideas and medical thinking see Fissell, *Vernacular Bodies*; on finances and organisation see Gorsky and Sheard, eds., *Financing Medicine*, and Smith, *Private Madhouses*.

19 Johannison, *Medicinens öga*; Moseng, *Ansvaret för undersåttenes helse*; Broberg, *Til at stwudera läkedom*.

20 Porter, *Health, Civilization and the State*; Uddenberg, *Lidande och läkedom*.

21 Dinges and Stolberg, 'Introduction,' 2.

care, bloodletting, cupping, and similar treatments. Secondly, there was the barber (Swe. *barberare*), whose task was the same as the previous category. Thirdly, barbers and 'bardskärare' were also a source for recruitment to the army. During the wars of the seventeenth century, these recruits were enlisted as 'fältskär,' barbers or 'bardskärare,' and their tasks in the army were similar to those of their civilian counterparts. In the discussion below, I will use the terms *barber* and *barber-surgeon* synonymously.

The guild privileges of barbers in Stockholm were confirmed at the end of the fifteenth century, and they were renewed in 1571 with regard to previously issued privileges which have not been preserved.[22] The privileges of 1571 and their confirmation were further steps in an ongoing institutionalisation and professionalisation of barbers' medical practice. At the same time, they were an expression of traditional corporate thinking, significant to society since the Middle Ages. Both aspects were represented in the privileges.

The privileges of 1571 consisted of twenty-eight paragraphs in which both duties to society and colleagues were articulated. For the individual barber, an affiliation to a guild was mandatory and a prerequisite for activities as a barber. It involved a fee, but also security in both professional practice and livelihood. Like the guilds' general function and order in the Middle Ages, it was clear that the directives of 1571 were aimed at limiting the number of practitioners in order to avoid over-establishment and injurious competition.[23] The number of master barbers was to be six and these masters must also be burghers of the city. However, the number of journeymen or assisting young boys was not regulated but was always to be decided in collaboration with the council members.

The feature of exclusivity was also clearly part of guild membership. Whoever wanted to enter the guild would have to offer proof of his honesty as well as completed years of schooling. No one would be allowed to enter a guild without having his competence tested.[24] Under the penalty of a fine, barbers could not have dealings with quacks ['lappare'] and others who unduly encroached on the barbers' duties, without running the risk of being treated as quacks themselves.[25] The guild's regulations thus protected not only the guild's competence in relation to outsiders, but also within the guild.

22 Lindström, *Skrå, stad och stat*, 86.

23 The original manuscript is preserved by Hagströmer Library in Stockholm. I have used a certified copy, preserved and provided by the National Archives (RA), in the archives of the Surgical society, *Kirurgiska societeten*. RA, *Kirurgiska societeten,* F I:8. § 1.

24 Ibid. §§ 3–4.

25 Ibid. § 23.

Moreover, several rules were in place to prevent barbers from competing with each other.[26] The guild organisation guarded and promoted domestic competence, although several of the barbers were from abroad, particularly from Germany. A foreign barber had to prove his skills for a longer period of time and more thoroughly than a native barber before inclusion in the guild, and his guild fee was also higher.[27]

Although affiliation was costly for the individual, the advantage gained was that the collective could jointly prevent unauthorised people from establishing themselves in the profession. Organisation into guilds also meant opportunities for the town authorities to increase their control of the guild members and their activities.[28] For example, the master of the guild was appointed by the town's authorities, on a yearly basis.[29] The guild organisation also meant opportunities for the guild to request protection of their competence by the authorities of the city. For example, it was stated that no quack should pretend 'artz' or to be a doctor, otherwise this would be punished by the city office.[30] It is clear that the privileges presented a broad and exclusive definition of a physician and that the guild perceived its role in healthcare as the most important thing to defend.

The guild was dependent on trust not only between colleagues, but also from trust upheld outside the guild. For that reason, there were rules for how the competence in the profession was to be maintained. If someone fell ill or was injured in connection with a barber's treatment, two of the city court judges, together with the masters in the guild, would carefully investigate and decide the question of guilt. If found guilty, the barber would lose his salary.[31] The guild organisation also cared for its members. Each individual barber contributed to a common fund that was to be used for needy guild members. This contribution was delivered every Sunday.[32]

The language in the privileges of 1571 was of an obvious masculine character. The paragraphs were generally addressed to 'he.' However, like other crafts, it was assumed that a barber conducted his activities within the framework of marriage and the household. This was expressed in several paragraphs. For example, if one of the colleagues' wives or children died, it

26 Ibid. § 5, 7.
27 Ibid. § 20.
28 Lindström, *Skrå, stad, stat*, 84.
29 RA, *Kirurgiska societeten* F I:8. § 2.
30 Ibid. § 26. The influence of the German language is obvious with the word *artz* (physician).
31 Ibid. § 10.
32 Ibid. § 14.

was assumed that members of the guild would attend the funeral.[33] It was also stipulated what would happen to the deceased's surviving wife and children. In the event of a barber's death, the widow would be allowed to maintain the activity as barber on the same terms as her deceased husband, as long as she could.[34] If the widow did not want to continue her deceased husband's work, she would sell the most precious thing she owned, that is, the office, to a candidate who was approved by both the city court judges and the guild.[35]

If both the barber and his wife died at the same time and left minor children, the guardian appointed was allowed to sell the office, although the consent of both the guild and the city council were required. When the children – if they were found to be honest – had grown up and settled in marriage, they had the opportunity to take up the profession of their deceased father and regain membership of the guild.[36] If a journeyman married a deceased master's wife or daughter, the guild would assist the journeyman in taking over the master's privileges upon passing the master's test.[37]

Apparently, a barber's activity was perceived as based on marriage and family. The first years of schooling took place within the family and were aimed at acquiring useful experiences. The system presupposed that male children would continue in their father's footsteps, while female children could eventually transfer master privileges to their spouses through marriage.[38] The privileges of 1571 emphasis on the importance of the household complicates the picture of the craft's gradual masculinisation process. They certainly do not state how the division of labour within the household was intended to be practised. However, the possibility, as stated in the privileges, for widows to take over the formal position of their deceased husbands, it is reasonable to believe that wives were familiar with the craft even when their husbands were alive.

What kind of healthcare did barbers offer? The privileges of 1571 are very vague. The only aspects mentioned are bloodletting, bandaging wounds, and applying patches and ointments.[39] The title of 'barber' indicates that cutting

33 Ibid. § 15.
34 Ibid. § 16.
35 Ibid. § 18.
36 Ibid. § 17.
37 Ibid. § 21.
38 The same system was practised by the burghers in medieval cities; see Jacbobsen, *Kvinder, kon og kobstadslovgivning*.
39 Ibid. §§ 9, 10, 23.

hair and grooming beards were also a part of the profession. Maybe it was so obvious that haircutting did not need to be explicitly formulated in the privileges. Given the other activities, which clearly specified different types of healthcare, cutting hair was perhaps seen as part of the healthcare of the time. Thus, the activities carried out by barbers were obviously diversified, but mainly concentrated to external and visible parts of the body. External healthcare as a barber's responsibility later became a guiding principle in the continued formalisation and institutionalisation of healthcare in Swedish society.

In 1680, the office of barbers in Stockholm was given expanded authority, including the supervision of barbers or barber-surgeons in the rest of the country. In 1695, Societas chirurgica, the Surgical Society (Swe. Kirurgiska societeten), was formed as the superior governing body for barber surgeons. In 1797, this became part of the above-mentioned Collegium Medicum. Bathers, who competed with barbers, also organised themselves in a guild (1657).[40] In practice, the activities of bathers and barbers were overlapping. Periodically during the seventeenth century, bathers worked as barber-surgeons at Danviken's hospital, for instance.[41]

When Collegium Medicum was established, regulations were issued that explicitly dismissed female knowledge of medicine. For example, a royal letter from 1684 complained that social practice did not conform to the directives issued in 1663. According to these instructions, medical remedies that were offered by strangers and ignorant people such as 'quacks and women' were forbidden. In the future, persons visiting the sick and practising medical care, were required approval by Collegium Medicum.[42] Thus women were by definition excluded due to their given ignorance. That provision was contrary to the privilege of a widow freely being able to continue the duties of her deceased husband, and it was also contrary to the basic corporative idea that the barber's enterprise took place within the framework created by marriage and the household.

On the surface of society, in terms of some regulations, a gradual masculinisation process in healthcare obviously occurred. However, the regulations did not prohibit a barber's wife from succeeding her deceased husband. Although the gender-coding in the language and implicit conditions were masculine, the family and household were obvious but not always articulated points of departure. Was this gradual masculinisation process also taking place below the surface of society?

40 Lindroth, *Svensk lärdomshistoria. Stormaktstiden*, 380, 383.

41 Lindberg, *Kirurgernas historia*, 34.

42 Hjelt, *Svenska och finska medicinalverkets historia*, 16.

Inside and outside the guild

From the seventeenth century onwards, it is clear that neither legal ordinances nor associations gave formal space to women, with the exception of the possibility of taking over a deceased husband's healthcare activities. This was a general trend in Europe. In practice, however, it was different. In the healthcare organisation that emerged in London at the turn of the century in 1600, for example, and in German cities during the seventeenth century, women continued to provide healthcare.[43] In practice, their importance was crucial for healthcare in several parts of Europe, although not officially recognised.[44] One area, close to a medical speciality but still independent, was however assessed to be mainly female: namely, midwifery. This speciality was also subject to regulations and training requirements as early as at the beginning of the eighteenth century. During this century, a division arose in childbirth practices in Sweden. Natural childbirth, which was probably most common, could still be taken care of by women. More technically complicated cases, which were more 'unnatural' and probably much less numerous, were to be taken care of by male obstetricians.[45]

Despite restrictions, it may be assumed that women in Sweden were engaged in healthcare activities, although this has not been systematically studied for the seventeenth and eighteenth centuries. The historian Kekke Stadin points out examples of women who, in the absence of barber-surgeons, were sanctioned by the city authorities to conduct the same kind of healthcare as barber-surgeons.[46] There are also examples of the authorities in the city of Stockholm commissioning a couple of particularly knowledgeable women to be responsible for the collection of herbs for medical use.[47] In her study of quackery in Sweden, Ling states that the meaning of the term 'quackery' varied between the eighteenth century and the end of nineteenth century. Moreover, accusations of quackery were few and far between in the eighteenth century. Ling also shows that the conflict between the different medical orientations, much emphasised in older research, was not actually that prominent.[48] An additional conclusion that can be drawn from her

43 Kinzelbach, 'Women and Healthcare,' 619–638.

44 Whaley, *Women and the Practice of Medical Care*, 131–149.

45 Vainio-Korhonen, *De frimodiga*; Paulsson Holmberg, *Onaturlig födelse*.

46 Stadin, 'Den gömda och glömda arbetskraften,' 309.

47 Thanks to Karin Sennefelt who let me share this information. Her observations originated from decisions made by the Collegium of Politii in Stockholm in the beginning of the seventeenth century.

48 Ling, *Kärringmedicin och vetenskap*, 113, 223.

study may thus be that women's medical practices were not considered sufficiently provocative for people to take legal action against licensed practitioners.

However, none of those accused of quackery were active as barber-surgeons. In studies of magic, some female healers emerge, but no barber-surgeons.[49] These studies show both women and men, who in various ways considered themselves able to cure diseases, appear in legally processed cases involving accusations of magic. However, the available evidence is strongly influenced by legal circumstances. Barbers were probably no more law-abiding than others, but their medical activities do not appear in this kind of source material, and nor does the medical care that was practised privately in people's own homes. Letters preserved from noble families show however that advice and instructions were frequently given to counteract colds, headaches, and other ailments.[50]

It is therefore very difficult to find sources that shed light on barbers' medical work and whether or not their wives and families were involved. A search for 'barber-surgeon' (Swe. *fältskär*) in the database *Gender and Work*, Uppsala University (*GaW*) gives only three search results. One result is a report from the local court in Snevringe in 1685. It explains the legal consequences of a fight on a farm in which the farmer defended himself with a knife against a soldier. Both the soldier and the farmer's wife were injured in the scuffle. The barber-surgeon Holger Klinth in Köping was sent for at night. He applied bandages to the wounds and was then sent back to Köping.[51] Another result includes a comment on how an army was put together, including barber-surgeons.[52] The third result concerns a case held in the town hall court in Örebro in the 1690s. The customs officer Lars Johansson accused a farmhand of letting his son to hit him on the head because the customs officer stopped them at the barrier. The barber-surgeon Lars Franck who was called in testified that it was only a flesh wound.[53]

These three cases reveal nothing about whether family and households were involved in the practical work. However, the cases suggest that 'fältskär' were mainly linked to cities and regiments and that their task was partly

49 Runesson, *Blod, kött och tårar*, 92–96.

50 Fries, *Märkvärdiga qvinnor*, 188; Rankin, *Panaceia's Daughters*.

51 *GaW*, case no. 10137. *GaW* includes thousands of fragmentary notices from different types of sources, primarily minutes from the local courts in rural areas, with information on how people in the past sustained and provided for themselves.

52 *GaW*, case no. 10344.

53 *GaW*, case no. 5944.

to assist the court in assessing the nature of possible injuries. A search for 'barber' gives a few more search results, a total of twelve, but with only a vague or no connection to medical activities.[54] Among the search results is also a population register from 1740, in which the inhabitants of the neighbourhood in Stockholm called Italy are listed together with their respective livelihoods. Dismissed non-commissioned officer Anders Rabé and his wife with their two children were said to support themselves as barbers.[55] No information however is given about the role of the household in the business.

Thus, we know with certainty that barbers continued with their work in the eighteenth century, at least in Stockholm, although we do not know anything about the organisation of that work. Outside the capital of Sweden, the digitised information is even more meagre. A search for the words 'fältskär' and 'barber' in the Swedish local history database, for which protocols from parishes in parts of southern and western Sweden have been transcribed and made searchable, gives no search results at all.[56]

On the surface and in the depths of society, a process of masculinisation among barber-surgeons seems to have been almost complete. However, there are some observations that can modify this image. One is the widow Sara Pfeil's petition to the Surgical Society in 1795.[57] She wrote that for many years her husband was a barber-surgeon in the mining district of Utö in the archipelago outside Stockholm, but that he had died from a stroke some years previously. She had become so distressed by his death that she had also suffered from a stroke. Despite her illness, she continued to pursue a career in medical care – she explicitly states that she learned the profession from her husband. She was now unable to manage any longer and asked for support. At the turn of the nineteenth century, it was clear that at least this barber-surgeon was running his business within the framework of a marriage and a household. However, if this was significant for barber-surgeons in general is still unclear.

Another example of the significance of a household may be illustrated by the regimental barber-surgeon Johan Fredrik Köllner. He was born in Kiel in 1721 but was already a barber-surgeon in the Kronoberg regiment at the age of twenty-one. In the war against Russia, 1741–1743, he served in the battle of

54 *GaW*, case nos. 5186, 8842.

55 *GaW*, case no. 15849.

56 *Svensk Lokalhistorisk Databas.*

57 RA, *Kirurgiska societetens arkiv.* Ämnesordnade handlingar, F1:5, Böneskrift från fältskärsenkan Sara Pfeil 1795.

Villmansstrand in 1741 and he participated in the entire Pomeranian war of 1757–1762. Köllner died at the age of sixty-six in 1784 and was succeeded by his son Bernhard Wilhelm Köllner, who later became a doctor of medicine.[58] A father and son working in the same field were completely in accordance with the tradition of the guilds, in which households and families were the basis for both work and training in the craft. First, knowledge was transmitted between fathers and sons, and additional medical experiences were gained elsewhere, often abroad. In this way, the craft was inherited, but formally only on the male side.

These examples raise some questions. Köllner was affiliated to the military, but conducted his work among civilians in the urban environment of Växjö, while Sara Pfeil was in an archipelago environment with no visible military or urban connection. Formally trained medical doctors and the guilds that were authorised to provide medical care, such as barbers, were mainly active in cities. The large number of hospitals (Swe. *lasarett*) that had been founded since the establishment of the Serafimer Hospital in Stockholm in 1752 were all located in cities.[59] On the other hand, most people lived in sparsely populated rural areas in eighteenth-century Sweden. Thus, the assumption must be that a majority of the population seldom or never came into contact with officially sanctioned healthcare. Perhaps opportunities were greater in rural areas for a more informally sanctioned medicine, with women as medical practitioners too. One can speculate that Sweden's second female doctor, Hedda Andersson, descended from a line of foremothers who had been active in the field for six generations. These women called themselves wound or fracture physicians, a term that covers approximately the same types of activity as those of barber-surgeons. In a similar manner to the guilds, in this case mothers and daughters passed down knowledge within the family through generations.[60]

The extent of the healthcare provided outside the officially sanctioned institutions and offices is impossible to estimate, especially in rural areas for which provincial doctors were responsible from the eighteenth century. These doctors had large districts and their task was mainly to prevent and combat recurring epidemics. In several of the provincial doctors' reports that have been preserved, they lament their own inadequacy. For example, the provincial doctor in Östergötland from 1754 to 1785, Johan Otto Hagström, wrote to the governor in 1755 and emphasised the shortage of doctors

58 Sjöberg, 'När sjukvården var militär,' 339–340.

59 Wawrinsky, *Sveriges lasarettsväsende*, Appendix I.

60 *Svenskt kvinnobiografiskt lexikon (SKBL)*, 'Hedda Albertina Andersson.'

who could easily have cured the diseases that were causing the poor to suffer premature death.[61] According to Hagström and his colleagues, the needs exceeded the individual physicians' practical possibilities. There is therefore reason to believe that the medical care offered outside the home was mostly of an informal nature with varying types of practitioners. Despite the fact that legislation had banned quackery since the 1660s and since then regulated who had the right to practise medical care, there were apparently practitioners who, if the legislation had been applied, would have been subject to legal proceedings. This suggests an interpretation that allows for the probable existence of an informal and unlicensed branch of healthcare, practised by both women and men, which was not sufficiently provocative that the authorities intervened. This interpretation corresponds with the perspectives and conclusions drawn by Ling in her above-mentioned study: 'Under normal circumstances physicians surprisingly often accepted quacks.'[62] The borders between disciplines and between licensed and unlicensed were thus blurred.

For instance, barber-surgeon Köllner, already mentioned above, reports how he cured the hunter Lars Bock's daughter from strange calluses and wounds from which she was suffering on both feet and hands. It appears that female medical practitioners had already been consulted but rejected. The parents' search for care was extended to the city of Växjö, where the mother took 'her wretched child' to the carpenter Vacan's wife, who 'was the most cunning medic I have ever seen, in Germany, Denmark, or Sweden.'[63]

Köllner took care of the little girl and several handwritten pages describe decoctions of various herbs that Köllner gave the girl for a long time – over a year. Of course, she finally regained her strength, her appetite returned, and even though at the end of the story there was still a wound as big as a 'buttonhole head' on her left arm, the girl was now restored.

Among the unlicensed healthcare practitioners in the eighteenth century were women, and although the authorities seemed to have tolerated them or been incapable of combating them, the formally competent and licensed healthcare practitioners were very critical in their condemnation. Their criticism was obviously coded as masculine, in which informal and unlicensed healthcare was coded as feminine. This would change, however, in the nineteenth century.

61 Hagström, *Johan Otto Hagströms brev*, 31.

62 Ling, *Käringmedicin och vetenskap*, 241.

63 RA, *Kirurgiska societetens arkiv*. Ämnesordnade handlingar, F1:3, bunt IX (RA).

Inclusion and hierarchy

The barber-surgeons of the eighteenth century were not a uniform category. A very influential group of barber-surgeons became specialised as formally trained surgeons.[64] Women played a significant role in this process. As mentioned earlier, complicated childbirths were to be taken care of by specialists, and this became a field for surgeons. This was true for two of the most renowned surgeons in Sweden during the eighteenth century: Olof af Acrel and Herman von Schützerkrantz. They shared a background as regimental barber-surgeons in the Svea Life Guards.[65] From a contemporary doctor's perspective at this time, surgery was only considered to be a simple handicraft, and not at all comparable to the sophisticated medical science of today.

However, when prestigious surgeons embraced the art of childbirth, they came to challenge the skills of a traditionally female professional group: the midwives. Thus, they followed the course founded by the medical doctor Johan von Hoorn in the late seventeenth century. Von Hoorn aimed to educate what he perceived as ignorant midwives and to stipulate what responsibilities they would have and what they would be prohibited from doing, such as using surgical instruments. In cases where complications occurred – unnatural childbirths – interventions of a more advanced kind were required, in practice operations performed exclusively by barber surgeons and doctors. However, the boundary between natural and unnatural birth was diffuse, which opened for a greater male involvement in childbirths.[66] An important background factor was an increased political interest in the growth of the population, where high infant mortality reduced the net population gain, and thus also an intensified interest in children and childhood.[67] Of less importance was the technological development.[68] The instruments used in complicated childbirths were knives and tongs that only barber-surgeons had the right to use.

Thus, obstetrics was practised by male surgeons, who were originally barber-surgeons. In that way, males gained control over the female body

64 Wolff, 'Kirurgerna och förnyelsen,' 470–496.

65 Sjöberg, 'Den lille grevens döda kropp,' 146–147.

66 Paulsson Holmberg, *Onaturlig födelse*, 116.

67 Paulsson Holmberg, *Onaturlig födelse*, 264–265.

68 The microscope had been invented, but its use in Sweden was rare until end of the nineteenth century. Caesarean sections have a long history, but not in Sweden; they were only undertaken as rare exceptions until the turn of the twentieth century. The suction bell did not come into use until the 1950s.

through a protected male activity. The losers were the female midwives. However, the process was not without conflicts or friction. The midwives wanted to maintain their monopoly on natural birth competence.[69] Despite repeated attacks from the medical doctors, they continued to have responsibility for the births of most pregnant women, the natural births. This is still the case. Royals and nobles, on the other hand, increasingly employed barber-surgeons and specialised doctors for so-called natural births. For example, Herman Schützerkrantz took part in delivering Queen Lovisa Ulrica in 1748 in her second childbirth. However, the resistance from midwives meant that he had to dress as a midwife of the time, which was also the case for his colleagues in France.[70] By dressing as a midwife, prevailing gender norms could in one sense be maintained.

Midwives and childbirth played a key role in the change during which obstetrics was invented and became surgery and thus a male field of activity.[71] At the same time, the midwives' demands to be permitted use forceps and other instruments during childbirth were part of a process that involved some traditional barber-surgeon activities leaving the domain of surgery and opening it for women. The status of surgery and obstetrics increased, while the status of vein care, wound care, and simple medical care decreased. Surgery and obstetrics became male fields of activity and vein care, wound care and simple medical care female. This development also applied to bathers, who from 1807 had to undertake the same surgical training as barber-surgeons. This resulted in several bathers becoming surgeons too.[72]

Fifty years later, in 1857, at a time when the guild system was being dissolved, qualifying as a bather also became a formal opportunity for women. However, bathers' formal education was abolished a few years later. This occurred in parallel to developments for barber-surgeons. The regulation for the practice of the barber-surgeons from 18 January 1861 states that vein care, cupping, enemas, dressing, shaving, bathing, splinting bone fractures, and exercising simpler wound care were the main areas of treatment. The same regulation established the qualifications required for practitioners. In addition to being of the approved age and good reputation, education as well as training as an apprentice were required. Both the education and the training were also available to women.[73]

69 Öberg, *Barnmorskan och läkaren*, 317.

70 Lundqvist, *Det svenska barnmorskeväsendet*, 15.

71 Compare Nilsson, *Det heta könet*, on the emergence of gynaecology.

72 Lindberg, *Kirurgernas historia*, 131.

73 *Svensk författningssamling*, 1861.

In 1861, the midwife Johanna Hedén qualified as Sweden's first female barber-surgeon. At the same time, nursing became a formally authorised profession for female healthcare practitioners. Through the 'Association for voluntary care of injured and sick in war' (Swe. Föreningen för frivillig vård av sårade och sjuka i fält), formal nursing education was an opportunity in Sweden from 1865. According to changes in legislation, healthcare was apparently at the beginning of a gender transformation. On a formal level, healthcare practitioners initiated a gradual feminisation. This is illustrated by the gender distribution among those who took their examinations and qualified as licensed barber-surgeons.

Table 1 shows that the profession of barber-surgeon continued to be male. An overwhelming majority of those who qualified were men. On the other hand, it appears that the number of women who qualified as barber-surgeons gradually increased and in the 1890s, when the education was terminated, the number of female barber-surgeons was just over half that of the male.

Table 1. Barber-surgeons examined, 1861–1900, women and men.

Time/Sex	Women	Men
1861–1870	2	24
1871–1880	1	22
1881–1890	14	36
1891–1900	35	66
Total	52	144

Table 8.1. Source: RA, Sundhetskollegium: Ombudsmannens övriga register och liggare, 1829–1877, 1852–1897. In general, the figures cannot be assumed to be complete. The total for 1861–1870 includes Johanna Hedén, whose degree is not listed in the volumes surveyed. Education in barber-surgery was terminated on 5 June 1896. The last candidates to qualify were examined in 1898.>

The legislative change can perhaps be explained by the fact that barber-surgeons' activities had fallen to such low status that they could be exercised by anybody, even women. Another explanation for the change may be changes in marriage patterns. Since the turn of nineteenth century, the number of formal marriages in Sweden had decreased (as was the case in other Western European countries, too). Unmarried men were of legal age and therefore had legal opportunities to support themselves, while unmarried women were prohibited from doing so. Unmarried women still needed to earn a living, however. Legislation responded to the situation and allowed unmarried women to come of legal age and have opportunities to support themselves.[74] A third explanation that ties in with the previous one lies in the fact that the role of marriage and the household for the barber-surgeon livelihood had changed. The large number of unmarried people in the society, at all levels, indicates this. However, there are other aspects that constitute complications. There must have been women who wanted to become barber-surgeons, but why did they not then attend nursing schools instead, for example? To some extent, these women provide a contradictory picture.

Johanna Hedén's life story shows that for her, the profession of midwife was a gateway. In her article in the *National Biographical Dictionary on Swedish Women* (Swe. *Svenskt kvinnobiografiskt lexikon, SKBL*), Pia Höjeberg points out that Hedén was the only person with healthcare experience at the copper mine and copper works in Huså. She was involved in taking care of the victims of several accidents and illnesses, not only in assisting women in childbirth, which was her formal employment. Therefore, Hedén felt compelled to improve her knowledge with a barber-surgeon training. There are other aspects as well, however. A few years after qualifying, Hedén moved south and took up the position of director on the Sahlgrenska childbirth ward in Gothenburg. In 1877, she married and resigned from her position since it was against the law for married women to be employed. However, her husband died in 1880, and Hedén then began an intensive community involvement in the cause of improving the working conditions of midwives. She was also active in the Fredrika Bremer Association which was an important part of the women's movement in Sweden.[75]

Community engagement and politics also interested one of the last people to be examined as a barber-surgeon in Sweden: Kerstin Hesselgren (1872–1962). She qualified as a barber-surgeon in 1895 and, in 1921, became one of the first five women members of the Swedish Parliament. Renée Frangeur, in her article about Hesselgren in *SKBL*, highlights both her deep social engagement, including being a member of the Fredrika Bremer Association, and her tomboyish nature as a little girl. Hesselgren nurtured a dream of becoming a doctor, which her father, himself a doctor, prevented.[76]

Several women dreamed of becoming doctors. In his article in *SKBL* about Amelina Sterky (1842–1922), Lindberg describes her desire to become a doctor. In her day, university studies in medicine were not yet possible for women. Sterky qualified as a barber-surgeon in 1889. She was also involved

74 Sjöberg, *Kvinnors jord, manlig rätt*, 175–179.

75 *SKBL*, 'Johanna Mariana Hedén.'

76 *SKBL*, 'Kerstin Hesselgren.'

in the Fredrika Bremer Association, which had a great impact on increasing the number of female barber-surgeons in the 1880s. The Association encouraged the idea of training nurses to become barber-surgeons so that they could later help the nation's population with basic healthcare and in the end compensate for the scarcity of doctors. Sterky was recruited as the principal for barber-surgeon education from 1894.[77]

Thus, some women barber-surgeons were deeply involved in women's issues, including political emancipation. Moreover, they were also emancipated in their everyday lives. They worked outside the home and acted independently in earning their livelihoods. The desire for independence is a further explanation why women who focused on the care of the sick chose the male barber-surgeon profession instead of a traditionally female nursing career. The hierarchically subordinate position of nurses in the few medical institutions that existed meant giving up opportunities for making a living and having a family, as well as the chance to organise their work themselves. More than other professions, nursing was a vocation for a whole lifetime, a mission in life, intended only for unmarried women. Married women were not permitted to be nurses. However, making a living as a barber-surgeon, with other medical activities as side lines, was possible for women, married and single. Such women transgressed the gender norms in their everyday emancipation throughout the nineteenth century when what is today called 'alternative' medicine was still part of 'normal' or 'school' medicine.

Conclusion: continuity and changes in gender norms

Barber-surgeons were seen as craftsmen in the sixteenth century, and as was the case with other craftsmen, they were organised in guilds that were family-based. Knowledge and skills were mainly transmitted from fathers to sons, since most guilds had mostly male members. However, it was assumed that wives had the knowledge and skills to take over their husbands' businesses if their husbands died. It is clear that neither Christianity nor the sixteenth-century Reformation had any intention of reducing the significance of this basic household organisation, which is obvious from the guild privileges issued towards the end of the sixteenth century. The language of the guilds was certainly masculine, and their rules were mainly aimed at male members of the guild. A few centuries later, the guild

77 *SKBL*, 'Amelina Mathilda Sterky.'

rules were abolished, and a career as a barber-surgeon became a licensed option for women. The Fredrika Bremer Association encouraged women to train as barbers. In this way, the organisation wanted to increase the number of healthcare practitioners so more people would have access to healthcare. However, the women who completed their studies and then worked as barber-surgeons were violating the current norms of femininity: they were self-employed and independent of a masculine market where healthcare was for sale, while the female nurses in institutional healthcare had a subordinate and dependent position.

How extensive the masculine healthcare market was is hard to estimate. Given that women in healthcare before the nineteenth century were largely invisible in the historical source material, whether they were active as barbers or in other functions, their significance cannot be expressed in quantitative terms. However, their invisibility was not total. They do occur from time to time in the sources. A reasonable, albeit hypothetical, conclusion is that women's professional involvement in healthcare activities has always existed, and that it has, for the most part, also been permitted, or at least tolerated. Women's involvement did not disturb the authorities and was therefore not documented. Sofia Ling's study shows, among other things, that the conflicts between licensed and unlicensed healthcare practitioners intensified during the second half of the nineteenth century, at least in the rhetoric and the intensity of their condemnation. This might mean that gender norms were also tightened so that there was less room for female entrepreneurship. A licence was required to engage in activities that had previously been undertaken without a licence.

This interpretation also suggests that barber-surgeons were now only allowed to carry out simple healthcare measures while formal, specialist surgery became a prestigious male development of the former barber's competence. A general conclusion is therefore that the everyday emancipation that individual female barber-surgeons might experience took place parallel to at least two processes. Firstly, licences and formal medical training meant that healthcare practitioners became visible and thus could also be controlled. Secondly, the authorities proclaimed a change in the content of the profession that made being a barber-surgeon less prestigious. Both processes coincided with the fact that the meaning of the notion health was about to change towards an approach where preventive measures were possible to secure future health. This change promoted a framework in which, to a large extent, the state authorities took responsibility for the subject's health.

Bibliography

Archival sources

Riksarkivet (the National Archives), (RA)
Kirurgiska societetens arkiv (Archives of the Surgical Society).
Sundhetskollegium.

Printed works

Johan Otto Hagströms, *Johan Otto Hagströms brev till collegium medicum 1755–1785*. Linköping: Östergötlands medicinhistoriska sällskap, 1993.
Svensk författningssamling, 1861.

Digitised works

Gender and Work (GaW), Uppsala University. https://gaw.hist.uu.se/. Accessed 21 June 2021.
Case no. 5186.
Case no. 8842.
Case no. 10137.
Case no. 10344.
Case no. 15849.
Svensk Lokalhistorisk Databas. https://www.lokalhistoria.nu/.

Literature

Berge, Anders. *Sjukvårdens underklass. Sjukvården i den kommunala fattigvården*. Umeå: Boréa, 2007.
Bergqvist, Johanna. *Läkare och läkande. Läkekonstens professionalisering i Sverige under medeltid och renässans*. Lund: Lund Studies in Historical Archaeology, 2013.
Brieger, Gert H. 'History of Medicine.' In *A Guide to the Culture of Science, Technology and Medicine*, edited by Paul T. Durbin, 121–194. New York: Free Press, 1980.
Broberg, Gunnar. *Til at stwudera läkedom: tio studier i svensk medicinhistoria*. Lund: Sekel förlag, 2008.
Crawford, Sally. 'The Nadir of Western Medicine? Texts, Contexts and Practice in Anglo-Saxon England.' In *Bodies of Knowledge. Cultural Interpretations of Illness and Medicine in Medieval Europe*, edited by Sally Crawford and Christina Lee, 41–51. Oxford: Archaeopress, 2010.
'Debate post.' *Läkartidningen* 103, no. 5 (2006): https://lakartidningen.se.

Dinges, Martin, and Michael Stolberg. 'Introduction.' In *Medical Practice, 1600–1900: Physicians and Their Patients*, edited by Martin Dinges, Kay Peter Jankrift, Sabine Schlegelmilch, and Michael Stolberg, 1–10. Leiden: Brill, 2016.

Fissell, Mary Elisabeth. *Vernacular Bodies: The Politics of Reproduction in Early Modern England*. Oxford: Oxford University Press, 2004.

Frangeur, Renée. 'Kerstin Hesselgren.' *Svenskt kvinnobiografiskt lexikon* (*SKBL*). https://skbl.se. Accessed 24 June 2021.

Fries, Ellen. *Märkvärdiga qvinnor*. Stockholm: Hierta, 1891.

Gorsky, Martin, and Sally Sheard, eds. *Financing Medicine: The British Experience since 1750*. London and New York: Routledge, 2006.

Hjelt, Otto E. A. *Svenska och finska medicinalverkets historia 1663–1812*, vol 1. Helsinki: Helsingfors central-tryckeri, 1891.

Höjeberg, Pia. 'Johanna Mariana Hedén.' *Svenskt kvinnobiografiskt lexikon* (*SKBL*). https://skbl.se. Accessed 24 June 2021.

Jacobsen, Grethe. *Kvinder, kon og kobstadslovgivning 1400–1600. Lovfaste Maend og aerlige Kvinder*. Copenhagen: Det Kongelige Bibliotek, Museum Tuscalanum, 1995.

Johannisson, Karin. *Medicinens öga. Sjukdom, medicin och samhälle – historiska erfarenheter*. Stockholm: Norstedt, 1990, 2013.

Johannisson, Karin, Ingemar Nilsson, and Roger Qvarsell. *Medicinen blir till vetenskap. Karolinska institutet under två århundraden*. Stockholm: Karolinska Institutet University Press, 2010.

Jütte, Robert. *Ärzte, Heiler und Patienten. Medizinischer Alltag in der Frühen Neuzeit*. Munich: Artemis und Winkler, 1991.

Kinzelbach, Annemarie. 'Women and Healthcare in Early Modern German Towns.' *Renaissance Studies* 28, no. 4 (2014): 619–638.

Lindberg, Bo S. 'Amelina Mathilda Sterky.' *Svenskt kvinnobiografiskt lexikon* (*SKBL*). https://skbl.se. Accessed 24 June 2021.

Lindberg, Bo S. *Kirurgernas historia. Om badare, barberare och fältskärer*. Uppsala: Uppsala universitet, 2017.

Lindroth, Sten. *Svensk lärdomshistoria. Frihetstiden*. Stockholm: Norstedt, 1978.

Lindroth, Sten. *Svensk lärdomshistoria. Stormaktstiden*. Stockholm: Norstedt, 1975.

Lindström, Dag. *Skrå, stad och stat. Stockholm, Malmö och Bergen ca 1350–1622*. Uppsala: Uppsala universitet, 1991.

Ling, Sofia. *Kärringmedicin och vetenskap. Läkare och kvacksalverianklagade i Sverige omkring 1770–1870*. Uppsala: Uppsala universitet, 2004.

Lundqvist, Birger. *Det svenska barnmorskeväsendets historia*. Stockholm, 1940.

Moseng, Ole Georg. *Ansvaret för undersåttenes helse 1603–1850*. Oslo: Universitetsforlaget, 2003.

Nilsson, Ulrika. *Det heta könet: gynekologin i Sverige kring förra sekelskiftet*. Stockholm: Wahlström och Widstrand, 2005.

Ohlander, Ann-Sofie. 'Hedda Andersson.' *Svenskt kvinnobiografiskt lexikon* (*SKBL*). https://skbl.se. Accessed 23 June 2021.

Oja, Linda. *Varken Gud eller natur. Synen på magi i 1600- och 1700-talets Sverige*. Eslöv: Symposium, 1999.

Paulsson Holmberg, Tove. *Onaturlig födelse. Johan von Hoorn och det obstetriska dilemmat 1680–1730*. Lund: Lunds universitet, 2017.

Porter, Dorothy. *Health, Civilization and the State: A History of Public Health from Ancient to Modern Times*. London and New York: Routledge, 1999.

Porter, Roy, ed. *The Cambridge History of Medicine*. Cambridge: Cambridge University Press, 2006.

Porter, Roy. *Health for Sale. Quackery in England 1660–1850*. Manchester: Manchester University Press, 1989.

Porter, Roy. *Patients and Practitioners. Lay Perceptions of Medicine in Pre-industrial Society*. Cambridge: Cambridge University Press, 1985.

Qvarsell, Roger, *Vårdens idéhistoria*. Stockholm: Carlsson, 1996.

Qvarsell, Roger, and Jan Sundin. 'The Social and Cultural History of Medicine and Health in Sweden.' *History and Philosophy of the Life Sciences* 17, no. 2 (1995): 315–336.

Radford Ruether, Rosemary. *Women and Redemption: A Theological History*. London: SCM Press, 1998.

Rankin, Alisha. *Panaceia's Daughters: Noble Women as Healers in Early Modern Germany*. Chicago: Chicago University Press, 2013.

Runesson, Anton. 'Blod, kött och tårar. Kroppslig erfarenhet i Sverige, ca 1600–1750.' PhD. diss., Stockholms universitet, 2021.

Sjöberg, Maria. *Kvinnors jord, manlig rätt. Äktenskap, egendom och makt i äldre tid*. Hedemora and Möklinta: Gidlunds, 2001.

Sjöberg, Maria. 'Den lille grevens döda kropp. Om rätt i 1700-talets medicin.' In *I utkanter och marginaler. 31 texter om kulturhistoria*, edited by Marianne Larsson, Anneli Palmsköld, Helena Hörnfeldt, and Lars-Eric Jönsson, 141–150. Stockholm: Nordiska museets förlag, 2015.

Sjöberg, Maria. 'När sjukvården var militär.' In *Allvarligt talat. Berättelser om livet*, edited by Maria Sjöberg, 335–352. Gothenburg: Makadam, 2018.

Smith, Leonard. *Private Madhouses in England, 1640–1815: Commercialised Care for the Insane*. Cham, Switzerland: Palgrave Macmillan, 2020.

Stadin, Kekke. 'Den gömda och glömda arbetskraften. Stadskvinnor i produktionen under 1600- och 1700-talen.' *Historisk tidskrift* 100, no. 3 (1980): 298–319.

Svenska Akademiens Ordbok (*SAOB*). Swedish Academy Dictionary, online: https://www.saob.se.

Tillhagen, Carl-Herman. *Folklig läkekonst*. Stockholm: LT, [1958] 1977.

Uddenberg, Nils. *Lidande och läkedom*. I. *Medicinens historia fram till 1800*. Stockholm: Fri Tanke, 2015.

Vainio-Korhonen, Kirsi. *De frimodiga: Barnmorskor, födande och kroppslighet på 1700-talet*. Helsinki: Svenska litteratursällskapet i Finland, 2016.
Wawrinsky, Richard. *Sveriges lasarettsväsende förr och nu*. Stockholm, 1906.
Whaley, Leigh. *Women and the Practice of Medical Care in Early Modern Europe, 1400–1800*. Palgrave Macmillan, 2011.
Wiesner, Merry E. 'Guilds, Male Bonding and Women's Work in Early Modern Germany.' *Gender & History* 1, no. 2 (1989): 125–136.
Wolff, Charlotta. 'Kirurgerna och förnyelsen av läkarvetenskapen i Finland 1751–1850.' *Historisk Tidskrift för Finland* 105, no. 4 (2020): 470–496.
Öberg, Lisa. *Barnmorskan och läkaren: Kompetens och konflikt i svensk förlossningsvård 1870–1920*. Stockholm: Ordfront, 1996.

About the Author

Maria Sjöberg is Professor of History at University of Gothenburg, Sweden. Her research focuses on gender history, primarily in the early modern period. She is the co-editor of *The National Biographical Dictionary of Swedish Women* (*SKBL*), the author of several books.

Epilogue: Epistemologies of Body and Soul: Considering the Early Modern and (Late) Modern History of Health

Helena Tolvhed

Abstract

The chapters of this volume demonstrate the protracted coexistence in the early modern era of a wide variety of medical knowledge regimes and practices for interpreting health and combating illness. In contrast, the modern medical paradigm, which consolidated its hegemonic authority in the first half of the twentieth century, understood health as primarily a concern of medical science and of the public sphere. However, the latter decades of the twentieth century saw a reemergence of alternative epistemologies and the growth of a multifaceted health market. The epilogue discusses comparisons, analogies, and contrasts between this era of 'late modernity' and the early modern era. Three main topics are discussed: the return of holistic new spirituality; the ideology of 'healthism' and the marketisation of health; and the emergence of fitness culture.

Keywords: health, healthism, fitness culture, alternative medicine, twenty-first century

Introduction

Today, as in the early modern era, great value is placed on the possession of health. This volume has uncovered health as a signifier of the good life in early modern society, understood in terms of happiness, tranquility, virtue, and prosperity. In this commentary chapter, I will move the discussion closer to our present time, focusing on the era from c. 1970 up until 'today,'

Eyice, M. and C. Forss (eds.), *Health and Society in Early Modern Sweden.*
Taylor & Francis Group 2024
DOI 10.5117/9789463724296_EPI

sometimes referred to as 'late modernity.' How can the high premium placed on achieving and maintaining health today be understood from the historian's perspective? Can health and wellness 'of body and soul' be likened – as has sometimes been suggested – to a secular religion, manifesting the virtuous (Swe. *dygdigt*) life, with places like the gym, the yoga studio, or the running track as temples of worship? Reflecting on the historically contingent nature of health, I will discuss the comparisons, analogies, and contrasts between the early modern and the late modern eras.

The chapters of this volume have demonstrated a great variance regarding the meaning and significance of 'health,' how it has been interpreted and imagined to be achieved and maintained. They have delineated the breadth of definitions of health, including mental, spiritual, and emotional dimensions, in the early modern era. Hence, this volume underlines the importance of historising and contextualising the conceptions and practices of health and illness as integrated in social relations, institutions, and the everyday lives of people from all social standings.

As Charlotta Forss and Mari Eyice point out in the introduction to this volume, the modern medical tradition grew from the consolidation of a Cartesian division between mind and body, stipulating a narrow definition of health focused on the well-being or disease of the biological body. This paradigm understood health as primarily a concern of medical science and the public sphere. In the first half of the twentieth century, the hegemonic authority of modern medicine and the medical profession were consolidated. However, as I will explicate in this epilogue, this absolute hegemony was challenged towards the end of the century.

This happened, I suggest, through a process of changing cultural and social norms combined with the commercialisation of health in the market-liberalised economy. This included the (re-)emergence of alternative and holistic conceptions of health and illness, tying into a growing and profitable market for health and wellness which in the 2000s has been further boosted through the rise of the internet and social media.

Another part of the health market which I will discuss in this epilogue is the field of exercise and fitness. The new fitness landscape that emerged from the early 1970s has been characterised, by critical scholars, as permeated by a 'healthist' discourse, where the responsibility for maintaining health is delegated to the individual citizen. This focus on illness prevention has been claimed to correspond to changes in the economic system, and political ambitions to cut welfare state spending in Sweden and elsewhere.

The reemergence of holistic conceptions of health

The chapters in this volume expose the rise of the scientific medical paradigm – resting on empirical observations, mathematics, chemistry, and biology – as a slow, uneven, and complex process of change. In Sweden, it was initiated through the emergence, from the late seventeenth century, of cultural and scientific societies and institutions. The authors point out the protracted coexistence and resilience of a wide variety of medical knowledge regimes and practices. The volume demonstrates the range of health practitioners drawing from and combining different knowledge regimes – both religious and 'worldly' – for interpreting health and combating illness.[1] For example, elements of Galenic/Hippocratic medicine, in which health was equal to a condition of balance between the four humours, remained influential in Swedish medicine until mid-nineteenth century.

The numerous healthcare practitioners in Sweden only slowly lost their status as formal medical professions as new scientific standards developed. By referring to science, the medical profession gained a monopoly over the business of healing and began to defend its newly won domain from around 1900. To uphold its authority, alternative medical ideas and practices were discarded as pseudoscience.[2] In recent decades, Sweden has seen a rise in the alternative medicine market, measuring higher levels compared to Denmark, Norway, and the US.[3] Historian of religion Ann-Christine Hornborg has characterised this development, starting in the 1980s, as both an expansion of the concept of health and an individualisation of health, leaving behind a previous socioeconomic and biomedical understanding of health.[4]

During the twentieth century, alternative medicine has continued to focus on well-being and the individual's own abilities to mobilise healing powers. The last half-century has seen a resurgence of and return to holistic ideas, emphasising mind–spirit balance, happiness, and well-being, in a way that is reminiscent of earlier medical paradigms and the broader conception of health elucidated in the chapters of this volume. These ideas and practices were boosted and revived with the New Age and counterculture movement of the 1960s and 1970s.

1 Hughes, 'Anthony Giddens,' 449.

2 Eklöf, *Från kvacksalveri*.

3 Hornborg, *Coaching*, 17. The most commonly used CAM methods in Sweden today, apart from chiropractic treatment and naprapathy, are medical massage, acupuncture, CAM medicines and relaxation techniques, such as medical yoga, *Komplementär och alternativ medicin och vård – säkerhet, kunskap, dialog*, Swedish Government Official Report (SOU) 2019:15.

4 Hornborg, *Coaching*, 17.

To further our understanding of these historical parallels and contrasts, inspiration can be drawn from research that discusses the development in health and wellness in terms of a reshaping of religious worlds rather than straightforward secularisation. Linda Woodhead and Paul Heelas have studied what they call a new spiritual holistic revolution in the West, characterised by the sacralisation of an individual's own search for meaning and an inner, spiritual, and authentic self. In this paradigm, spirituality is central, though traditional religion with its teachings and traditional places of practice is not highly valued.[5]

Other researchers have emphasised how markets have been built around the teachings and facilitation of self-development and self-improvement, appropriating and commercialising the spirit of 1960s and 1970s New Age and counterculture.[6] Furthermore, as pointed out by Raka Shome, the Western world's consumption of Eastern body-cultural traditions should also be placed in a context of global power relations. This discussion on health should also note the gender dimension, with women being central as consumers, entrepreneurs, and service workers in the field of wellness. The Eastern influenced 'wellness' trend, including yoga, massage, and spa treatments, has mainly been directed towards providing recreation to white, Western, and financially well-off women.[7]

Today's landscape of health practices is characterised by increasing medical pluralism, including chiropractic treatment, naprapathy, yoga, alternative medicine, massage- and stress management-therapies, acupuncture, qi gong, reiki healing, homeopathy, herbal medicine, mindfulness, and various dietary prescriptions for restoring and keeping health. Products and services in health, wellness, and fitness are commercially provided by a plethora of actors and (semi-)professionals.

Today, it is not necessarily a lack of access to academic and clinical medical treatments that makes people turn to various alternative strategies (although this can also be a factor). Complementary and alternative medicine (CAM) is now a major part of the healthcare system in all modern, complex societies, integrated in a consumer culture and economy where the individual consumer is offered 'freedom of choice.' The CAM market and the 'orthodox' healthcare sector both have undergone significant marketisation, underpinning the integration and normalisation of CAM-actors in healthcare

5 Heelas and Woodhead, *The Spiritual Revolution*.

6 McGee, *Self-Help; Inc.*; Carrette and King, *Selling Spirituality*. On Swedish spirituality in the twentieth century, see Thurfjell, *Det gudlösa folket*.

7 Shome, *Diana and Beyond*.

as providers of services and products enter this expanding market.[8] The trend toward alternative medicine has been officially recognised by the World Health Organization (WHO). The organisation's first strategy of traditional and complementary medicine was developed in the beginning of the twenty-first century and has now been adopted by the WHO Traditional Medicine Strategy 2014–2023.[9]

Hence, the situation demonstrates some similarities with how early modern people drew on health advice and treatments from different groups of actors and knowledge regimes. For example, sauna baths have made a widespread comeback, imagined and marketed as self-care, relaxation, and socialisation. Bathing, including mineral baths and mud packing treatments at spas and health resorts, has continued to be used for health purposes and is thought to benefit those suffering from joint and muscle pain as well as skin diseases.

'Healthism' and the marketisation of health from the 1970s

A growing research field has described how health and healthiness has emerged not only as an ideal, but also as a responsibility of the individual in the late twentieth century. These developments must, of course, be historicised and understood as entrenched within political, social, and economic contexts. Already in 1980, Robert Crawford identified an emerging ideology of 'healthism' as emblematic for his own time. Having health and a fit body, he argued, have become lifestyle markers and metaphors for morality and a good life. In this ideology, subjects are constructed as autonomous agents responsible for their own well-being, without consideration of the impact of social and economic determinants. Health has, according to Crawford, become a 'super value,' implicating not only the absence of illness but also the presence of happiness, a sense of self, the ability to function, and evidence of work-life productivity. The underlying assumption here is that ill-health is (largely) preventable.[10]

In a welfare state such as Sweden, the rise of neoliberalism since the late 1970s has meant a fundamental shift. Historical research has pointed out how health policy and discourse in Sweden began to transform from the

8 Collyer, 'The Corporatisation'; Tovey, Easthope, and Adams, 'Introduction.'

9 Swedish Government Official Report (SOU) 2019:15, 236.

10 Crawford, 'Healthism,' 365–388; Peterson and Lupton, *The New Public Health*; Rose, 'Government and Control,' 321–339, 337.

all-embracing modern welfare state towards a more individualised direction from the 1970s. The authorities' way of speaking to and about the citizen increasingly emphasised the importance of individual lifestyle and the prevention of ill-health. The idea that individuals should take responsibility for their own health fitted well with efforts to cut government spending in the welfare sector, and neoliberal ideas that restructured economies all over the world.[11] The possession of health and a fit body have also become prominent as requirements and competitive advantages in an increasingly demanding, insecure, and deregulated working life.[12]

The concept of healthism should be understood as closely related to Michel Foucault's theoretical concept of biopolitics, a regulating regime where human life is managed through knowledge and power, and the related processes of shaping new forms of subjectivities.[13] Foucault argued that the character of biopolitics changed during the twentieth century, from the disciplinary regimes of families, hospitals, schools, and factories, towards more sophisticated techniques of governing. In late modern consumer culture, power primarily works through stimulation and internalised self-monitoring, influencing the way people think, feel, and perceive.[14]

The emphasis on individual responsibility is central to specific forms of governance in advanced liberal – or neoliberal – democracies since the end of the twentieth century. Norms regarding what constitute acceptable choices mean that citizens regulate themselves from within. The citizen is made into a consumer who supposedly makes 'free' choices in the markets of education, work, housing, and various consumer goods and services. The consequences of incorrect 'choices' must be the responsibility of each citizen.[15] In the new modes of regulating health, individuals are discursively addressed on the assumption that they *want to be healthy* – not least due to the synonymous use of 'healthiness' and 'happiness' – and directed to seek out the ways of living most likely to promote their own health.

11 Palmblad and Eriksson, *Kropp och politik*; Johannisson, *Kroppens tunna*; Olsson, *Drömmen om*; Metzl, 'Introduction.' Neoliberal ideology has influenced the Nordic welfare societies, following debates on 'bureaucratic' state systems, and 'efficient' competition models, and has been introduced to Nordic political sphere since the late twentieth century. Ivarsson Westerberg, Waldemarson, and Östberg, eds., *Det långa 1990-talet*.

12 Björklund, *Constituting*; Cederström and Spicer, *The Wellness Syndrome*; Crawford, 'Healthism'; Dworkin and Wachs, *Body Panic*; Petersen and Lupton, *The New Public Health*.

13 See also the introductory chapter in this volume.

14 Foucault, *Discipline and Punish*; Foucault, 'Body/Power.'

15 Rose, *Powers of Freedom*. See also discussion on the 'empowered patient' norm and policies such as the British 'Expert Patient' programme, introduced by the Blair government in 1999, in Gabe and Almeida, 'Anthony Giddens: Structuration.'

Correspondingly, a multifaceted health market expanded during the last decades of the twentieth century, exploiting the commercial potential in the plethora of medical ideas and practices. In the light of the chapters of this volume, some resemblances to the early modern situation can be noted. The (re-)emerging, multifaceted health market encompasses alternative epistemologies which contemplate health and the treatment of illness in a way that, at least to some extent, challenges and dissolves former monopolies and the supreme authority of modern scientific medicine, as well as the power of pharmaceutical industries.[16]

Today, however, products, diets, supplements, and various forms of exercise, mindfulness, and yoga are presented as matters of personal choice and taste, even as aspects of identity. Experts instruct us as to how to be healthy, advertisers project the appropriate actions and fulfilments, and entrepreneurs develop a market for health.[17] Dietary programs and trends appear, sometimes offering contradictory advice on how to regulate body weight and/or achieve or maintain health and fitness through dietary practises. These frequently appear as complements, or even alternatives, to the recommendations of scholarly medicine.

In this expanding health market, new and still-growing professions have emerged in the form of, for example, health coaches and personal trainers. Another part of this trend is the rise in books and other media – magazines, newspapers, online media, podcasts – that are circulating the latest advice and ideas of diet and exercise, news of health-related studies, and changing trends in well-being. Furthermore, electronic self-monitoring devices provide the user with data on the inner functions of the body. Consumers willing and able to buy these products can monitor bodily functions and set goals and quotas in order to maximise their potential, without venturing near a doctor's office.

Hence, paralleling the early modern era, a situation of competing epistemologies has arisen. Some scholars have argued that biomedicine's appeal is waning and identify causes such as the increasing emphasis on consumption – rather than production – in the postmodern economy, shifting attitudes towards science, the commodification of the new attitudinal dispositions and the declining power of the state to influence the market. In this situation, consumers pursue the treatments that they believe in, to the extent that these are available and affordable to them.[18]

16 Hughes, 'Anthony Giddens,' 439.

17 Rose, *Powers of Freedom*, 86–87.

18 Tovey, Easthope, and Adams, 'Introduction.'

Fitness culture, appearance, and identity

Whereas the scientific paradigm of the modern era focused on measuring the statistics of the body, health today also denotes a distinctly visual element, and the visibility of health practices. This section will highlight the entanglements of health and beauty, working in both directions, as the slim, 'toned,' and good-looking body emerged as the ultimate symbol of health. Looking healthy and fit has become a visual sign of youth, success, and the discipline needed to perform health.

With the jogging wave of the 1970s and the gym and fitness trend of the 1980s, a new landscape of physical culture emerged. An increasingly globalised and commercialised fitness industry emerged on a broader scale, with an agenda largely set by private operators. Arnold Schwarzenegger went from muscle hero to action film Hollywood star during the 1980s, giving the bodybuilding sport unprecedented popularity. Weight training moved from small basement gyms into fresh and bright new fitness clubs, marketed towards affluent segments of society.

In Sweden, the expanding commercial health industry has challenged and transformed a previous public health regime characterised by strong state control and close ties to the national sports movement (*Riksidrottsförbundet*). As traditional sports and play have been partly replaced by new forms of exercise, the Swedish sport movement has lost ground to privatised market. Trending new forms of exercise, clothing and other products appear as increasingly entrenched in everyday and popular culture.[19]

In the 1980s, actress Jane Fonda pioneered the 'workout' home video, building a massive fitness empire. In Sweden, Susanne Lanefelt led the breakthrough of home training and fitness culture more generally, with the TV show *Gymping*, broadcast from 1983 to 1987. In this burgeoning culture of fitness and exercise, women became central consumer targets and the physically active, fit, and muscularly 'sculpted' female emerged as a new normative ideal.[20] This stands in stark contrast to an earlier history in which the practising of many sports, well into the twentieth century, was considered incompatible with conceptions of respectable femininity and

19 McKenzie, *Getting Physical*; Smith Maguire, *Fit for Consumption*; Andreasson and Johansson, *The Global Gym*; Tolvhed and Hakola, 'The Individualization of Health.' The gym and fitness industry has been expanding steadily, mainly in the Western world but also in countries such as Brazil, Japan, and China. IHRSA (The Global Health and Fitness Association) *Global Report 2020* concludes: 'Worldwide, industry revenue totaled US$96.7 billion in 2019, as more than 184 million members belonged to nearly 210,000 health and fitness facilities.'

20 Dworkin and Wachs, *Body Panic*.

women frequently were warned of the physically and mentally harmful and masculinising effects of (especially competitive) sports and strenuous physical activities.[21] It is, furthermore, interesting to consider the rise of female entrepreneurs and influencers in today's health field against a historical background where increasing emphasis on formal training meant masculinisation. This volume offers ample examples of how gender norms show flexibility, over time and in relation to changing conditions.

Today's popular cultural and commercial body norms and ideals appear closely associated with diet and exercise practices, and constructed through various intersections between gender, class, and race/ethnicity. Female models used to represent 'health' – marketing products, clothing, or services mainly to an affluent middle class – are conventionally beautiful, smiling, white, and predominately thin rather than obviously muscular. This limits the destabilising potential of the 'fit' woman.[22]

The body is constructed as a project, in need of constant maintenance and open to reconstruction and improvement – it is forever unfinished.[23] When the 'healthy' body is perceived as a reflection of self-control and a 'healthy' inner world of the subject, the unhealthy body is subsequently read as a moral and aesthetic personal failure.[24] Lifestyle norms are disseminated in leisure time as well as in working life. Whereas the emblematic (male) 'boss' of the industrial era was traditionally imagined as the manufacturer, a perhaps slightly corpulent capitalist dressed in elegant clothes symbolising well-being and prosperity, today's leaders (still usually male, but conceivably female) would rather be thought of as Lycra-clad and participating in demanding athletic events such as the 'Swedish classic,' marathon, or triathlon. Top managers are expected to inspire their employees to perform not only at work, but also in healthy living and exercise.[25]

Conclusion: coexisting epistemologies and precarious prospects

This volume offers ample examples of practitioners promoting their own agenda in the field of health and illness in the early modern period. The

21 Cahn, *Coming on Strong*; Hargreaves, *Sporting Females*; Tolvhed, *På damsidan*.

22 Dworkin and Wachs, *Body Panic*; Tolvhed, *På damsidan*, ch. 7

23 Shilling, *The Body*, 4–8, 199–200.

24 Dworkin and Wachs, *Body Panic*; LeBesco, 'Neoliberalism, Public Health' 153–164; Petersen and Lupton, *New Public Health*, 68–69.

25 Björklund, *Constituting*; Cederström and Spicer, *The Wellness Syndrome*; Petersen and Lupton, *The New Public Health*.

chapters demonstrate how the early modern period was set in both an ancient tradition and folk heritage, in addition to the Christian worldview. Health was understood as tranquility, happiness, virtue, and prosperity, well beyond the medical sphere, and thought to be maintained through daily practices, routines, and various rituals.

I have argued for the interpretation that the last fifty-year period has witnessed something of a re-emergence in Western culture and society of a broader concept of health as a good life. Health and (the appearance of) a healthy lifestyle has emerged as, if not a secular religion, as something of a super-value, and a manifestation of a virtuous life. Furthermore, in this culture, the 'fit' body is presented as a prime visual symbol of success and ability to perform at work. Hence, health – or rather, its imagined forms and expressions – emanates as a virtue in itself, as *the* virtue, rather than as a means to some other end, or to reward in the afterlife. The purpose of the healthy lifestyle is the long and healthy life itself, in what immunologist and renowned writer Barbara Ehrenreich has named a fundamental 'quest for control' over life and death.[26]

The 'healthist' discourse directs the responsibility for maintaining health and preventing illness onto the individual, who may be subject to suspicion of having failed in this duty. With the increasing demand for self-management, critics have noted a growing 'health stress' and body fixation, and questioned the current development where the employee's health has become a concern for employers and means to recruit workers in today's competitive and 'flexible' labour market.[27] In a constant mode of self-improvement, this unfinishedness feeds into the growing field of knowledge and technical expertise for altering the shape, appearance, and performance of the body.[28] The emphasis on consumption, of course, makes this a lifestyle that is not available to less affluent segments of society.

As Zygmunt Bauman has discussed, current discourses of life, health, and death seem permeated by the late modern fantasy of defeating the limitations and conditions of human life. Everything, including disease, aging, the limits of ecological systems, and even death, can be managed and overcome.[29] In the late twentieth century, the focus has shifted from social citizenship with obligations deriving from membership in a collective

26 Ehrenreich, *Natural Causes*, xiv.

27 Cederström and Spicer, *The Wellness Syndrome*; Ehrenreich, *Natural Causes*, 63.

28 Bordo, *Unbearable Weight*; Petersen and Lupton, *The New Public Health*; Shilling, *The Body and Social Theory*.

29 Bauman, *Consuming Life*.

body to an individualistic discourse emphasising personal gains and making informed consumer choices. Wendy Brown has formulated what she calls a 'post-political' state: 'The model neo-liberal citizen is one who strategises for her/himself among various social, political and economic options, not one who strives with others to alter or organise these options.'[30] People have lost faith in politics, and the change that appears to be available is not political – that is, collective action for social change – but instead personal change in life circumstances and care for one's own spiritual and physical health.[31]

While the standing of modern scientific medicine is still strong, there exists today – as I have elucidated in this epilogue – a flourishing field of alternative, competing prescriptions on how to maintain health and cure illness. Social media blogs, magazines, and the book market are abundant with advice and self-help literature that are frequently unconfirmed by solid scientific research. However, when health and illness are – as is the perspective of this volume – regarded as historically contingent phenomena, the 'healthist' discourse is not a given; it is changeable, and, furthermore, it is not all-encompassing in our present culture. There is room for political debate, activism for societal change, and alternative lifestyles.

It remains to be seen what new conceptualisations of health await in the near future. It is plausible that the Covid-19 pandemic will – when viewed by future historians – contribute to a strengthening of medical authority (although those resisting this authority certainly made their voices heard during the pandemic, too). Even more momentous, the climate crisis threatens to undermine the fundamentals of our existence on this earth. In the 2020s, WHO identifies climate change as the single biggest health threat facing humanity: if we are to make the shift towards a broader understanding of health, we must also promote sustainability and respect for planetary boundaries.

Bibliography

Literature

Andreasson, Jesper, and Thomas Johansson. *The Global Gym: Gender, Health and Pedagogies*. Basingstoke, Hampshire: Palgrave Macmillan, 2014.

Bauman, Zygmunt. *Consuming Life*. Cambridge: Polity, 2007.

30 Brown, *Edgework*.

31 Mouffe, *On the Political*; McGee, *Self-Help, Inc.*

Björklund, Erika. *Constituting the Healthy Employee? Governing Gendered Subjects in Workplace Health Promotion*. Umeå: Umeå universitet, 2008.

Bordo, Susan. *Unbearable Weight: Feminism, Western Culture, and the Body.* Berkeley: University of California Press, 1993.

Brown, Wendy. *Edgework: Critical Essays on Knowledge and Politics*. Princeton, NJ: Princeton University Press, 2005.

Cahn, Susan K. *Coming on Strong: Gender and Sexuality in Twentieth-Century Women's Sport*. New York: Harvard University Press, 1995.

Carrette, Jeremy R., and Richard King. *Selling Spirituality: The Silent Takeover of Religion*. London: Routledge, 2005.

Cederström, Carl, and André Spicer. *The Wellness Syndrome*. Cambridge: Polity, 2015.

Collyer, Fran. 'The Corporatisation and Commercialisation of CAM.' *The Mainstreaming of Complementary and Alternative Medicine: Studies in Social Context*, edited by Philip Tovey, Gary Easthope, and Jon Adams, 81–101. London: Routledge, 2004.

Crawford, Robert. 'Healthism and the Medicalization of Everyday Life.' *International Journal of Health Services* 10, no. 3 (1980): 365–388.

Drakman, Annelie. *När kroppen slöt sig och blev fast: Varför åderlåtning, miasmateori och klimatmedicin övergavs vid 1800-talets mitt*. Uppsala: Uppsala universitet, 2018.

Dworkin, Shari L., and Faye Linda Wachs. *Body Panic: Gender, Health, and the Selling of Fitness*. New York: New York University Press, 2009.

Ehrenreich, Barbara. *Natural Causes: Life, Death and the Illusion of Control*. London: Granta, 2018.

Ekenstam, Claes. *Kroppens idéhistoria. Disciplinering och karaktärsdaning i Sverige 1700–1950*. Hedemora: Gidlund, 2006.

Eklöf, Motzi. *Från kvacksalveri till alternativmedicin: Sammanfattning av Alternativmedicinkommitténs utredning*. Stockholm: Allmänna förlaget, 1989.

Foucault, Michel. 'Body/Power.' In *Michel Foucault: Power/Knowledge*, edited by Colin Gordon. New York: Pantheon Books, 1980.

Foucault, Michel. *Discipline and Punish: The Birth of the Prison*, 109–133. New York: Pantheon Books, 1977.

Gabe, Jonathan, and Joana Almeida. 'Anthony Giddens: Structuration, Drug Use, Food Choice and Long-Term Illness.' In *The Palgrave Handbook of Social Theory in Health, Illness and Medicine*, edited by Fran Collyer, 424–438. Basingstoke: Palgrave Macmillan, 2015.

Gilman, Sander L. *Fat. A Cultural History of Obesity*. Cambridge Polity, 2008.

Hargreaves, Jennifer. *Sporting Females: Critical Issues in the History and Sociology of Women's Sports*. London: Routledge, 1994.

Heelas, Paul, and Linda Woodhead. *The Spiritual Revolution: Why Religion Is Giving Way to Spirituality*, Malden: Blackwell, 2005.

Hornborg, Anne-Christine. *Coaching och lekmannaterapi: En modern väckelse?* Stockholm: Dialogos, 2012.

Hughes, Kate. 'Anthony Giddens: The Reflexive Self and the Consumption of Alternative Medicine.' In *The Palgrave Handbook of Social Theory in Health, Illness and Medicine*, edited by Fran Collyer, 439–454. Basingstoke: Palgrave Macmillan, 2015.

Ivarsson Westerberg, Anders, Ylva Waldemarson, and Kjell Östberg, eds. *Det långa 1990-talet: När Sverige förändrades*. Umeå: Boréa, 2014.

Johannisson, Karin. *Kroppens tunna skal: Sex essäer om kropp, historia och kultur*. Stockholm: Norstedt, 1997.

Komplementär och alternativ medicin och vård – säkerhet, kunskap, dialog. Swedish Government Official Report (SOU) 2019:15.

LeBesco, Kathleen. 'Neoliberalism, Public Health, and the Moral Perils of Fatness.' *Critical Public Health* 21, no. 2 (2011): 153–164.

McGee, Micki. *Self-Help, Inc.: Makeover Culture in American Life*. Oxford: Oxford University Press, 2005.

McKenzie, Shelly. *Getting Physical: The Rise of Fitness Culture in America*. Lawrence: University Press of Kansas, 2013.

Metzl, Jonathan. 'Introduction: Why Against Health?' In *Against Health: How Health Became the New Morality*, edited by Jonathan Metzl and Anna Kirkland, 1–10. New York: New York University Press, 2010.

Mouffe, Chantal. *On the Political*. London: Routledge, 2005.

Olsson, Ulf. *Drömmen om den hälsosamma medborgaren: Folkuppfostran och hälsoupplysning i folkhemmet*. Stockholm: Carlsson, 1999.

Palmblad, Eva, and Bengt Erik Eriksson. *Kropp och politik: Hälsoupplysning som samhällsspegel från 30-tal till 90-tal*. Stockholm: Carlsson, 1995.

Peterson, Alan, and Deborah Lupton. *The New Public Health. Health and Self in the Age of Risk*. London: Sage, 1996.

Rose, Nikolas. 'Government and Control.' *British Journal of Criminology* 40, no. 2 (2000): 321–339.

Rose, Nikolas. *Powers of Freedom. Reframing Political Thought*. Cambridge: Cambridge University Press, 1999.

Shilling, Chris. *The Body and Social Theory*. London: Sage, 1993.

Shome, Raka. *Diana and Beyond: White Femininity, National Identity, and Contemporary Media Culture*. Champaign: University of Illinois Press, 2014.

Smith Maguire, Jennifer. *Fit for Consumption: Sociology and the Business of Fitness*. Abingdon: Routledge, 2007.

Stearns, Peter N. *Fat History. Bodies and Beauty in the Modern West.* New York: New York University Press, 1997.

The 2020 IHRSA Global Report, The Global Health and Fitness Association, 2020. https://www.ihrsa.org/publications/the-2020-ihrsa-global-report.

Thurfjell, David. *Det gudlösa folket: De postkristna svenskarna och religionen.* Stockholm: Molin & Sorgenfrei, 2015.

Tolvhed, Helena. *På damsidan. Femininitet, motstånd och makt i svensk idrott 1920–1990.* Gothenburg: Makadam förlag, 2015.

Tolvhed, Helena, and Outi Hakola. 'The Individualization of Health in Late Modernity.' In *Conceptualising Public Health: Historical and Contemporary Struggles over Key Concepts*, edited by Johannes Kananen, Sophy Bergenheim, and Merle Wessel, 190–203. Oxford: Routledge, 2018.

Tovey, Philip, Gary Easthope, and Jon Adams. 'Introduction.' In *The Mainstreaming of Complementary and Alternative Medicine: Studies in Social Context*, edited by Philip Tovey, Gary Easthope, and Jon Adams, 1–8. London: Routledge, 2004.

About the Author

Helena Tolvhed is Reader in History at Stockholm University. Her research includes work on twentieth-century understandings of health and the role of gender in modern sport.

Index

For Product Safety Concerns and Information please contact our EU representative GPSR@taylorandfrancis.com
Taylor & Francis Verlag GmbH, Kaufingerstraße 24, 80331 München, Germany

www.ingramcontent.com/pod-product-compliance
Ingram Content Group UK Ltd.
Pitfield, Milton Keynes, MK11 3LW, UK
UKHW022131190926
475702UK00013B/1757
9781041180784